Banish Back Pain the Pilates Way

Other books by Anna Selby:

Pilates for Pregnancy
Pilates for a Flat Stomach

Anna Selby
Foreword by Clare Fone MCSP, SRP

Banish Back
Pain the
Pilates Way

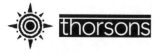 thorsons

Thorsons
An Imprint of HarperCollins*Publishers*
77–85 Fulham Palace Road,
Hammersmith, London W6 8JB

The website address is www.thorsonselement.com

-ᛜ- thorsons™

and *Thorsons* are trademarks of
HarperCollins*Publishers* Limited

First published 2003

10 9 8 7 6 5 4 3 2 1

A catalogue record for this book
is available from the British Library

ISBN 0 00 714126 2

Photography © Guy Hearn
Text illustration by PCA Creative

The publishers wish to thank the models, Deborah Henley and
Mario F. Perez at The Pilates Room, for all their help with the photo shoot.
For more information on The Pilates Room, see the Resources section.

Printed and bound in Great Britain by
Martins The Printers Ltd, Berwick upon Tweed

Contents

Foreword

The number of back pain sufferers is growing. In my clinic, the majority of my patients complain of a gradual onset of back pain. This is often due to poor posture, sustained both at work and at home. The only way good posture is maintained is by strengthening the postural muscles through consistently correct use. Our present lifestyles do nothing to maintain good posture.

A baby naturally develops perfect posture. However, this is easily lost during childhood as children slump in front of the television and while using computer games. As adults, we spend increasing amounts of time at a computer, driving cars and generally leading rather sedentary lives. Regular exercise is therefore vital to maintain muscle strength. Pilates, yoga and swimming are key all-round exercise approaches. They assist in promoting good posture and also in balancing the one-sided muscle development that some sports often create.

Healthy tissues need oxygen. We need to breathe as efficiently and effectively as possible to get the maximum amount of oxygen into the lungs, from where it is then circulated around the body. Most of us shallow breathe and never deep breathe into the base of the lungs, unless we are doing vigorous exercise. Pilates teaches us to breathe properly. It works all the postural muscles, improving pelvic stability and enabling correct use of the joints. Pilates is here to stay.

Pilates exercises should be part of our lifestyle. By incorporating the exercises into our daily activities we are conscious of how we hold ourselves and in time, this becomes an everyday habit. This book, with its well-written, clear and easy-to-follow exercises, is the ideal means of achieving this.

Put simply, if you want to look straighter, slimmer, more confident and fitter – do Pilates!

CLARE FONE MCSP, SRP, CERT. HEALTH ED
THE WESTMINSTER PHYSIOTHERAPY CENTRE

Introduction

Back pain has reached epidemic proportions. It is one of the most common causes of lost working days, as well as of visits to the doctor. Back pain is reported by 60 % of people at some time in their lives, and the costs of medical treatment and lost production to business amount to billions annually.

The problem is much more than financial, however. Back pain is a debilitating condition. If you have severe back pain, normal life comes to a complete halt. You cannot do any of your normal activities, you probably need to take powerful painkillers simply to endure the pain and – at least at first – you are likely to be reduced to lying in bed, suffering. On top of all this, many people don't take back pain particularly seriously, especially if it is difficult to pinpoint a specific discernible, cause – and, far from receiving any sympathy, you may end up accused of being 'lazy' or malingering.

Back pain is all too real to the huge numbers of people who suffer from it. But there is hope: many health care professionals – doctors, physiotherapists, osteopaths and chiropractors – believe that much back pain is avoidable. Rather than focusing on external problems, such as injury, sporting accidents, lifting heavy weights, they believe that by concentrating on making your back as strong and flexible as possible, you will make it much less vulnerable to pain and problems.

This book offers a Pilates approach to the problem. Initially developed as a system to help the injured of the First World War, its creator, Joseph Pilates, began by using a system of strings and pulleys so that those who were confined to their beds could still keep their muscles toned without risking any further injury. Although much developed and extended by Pilates and others since those early days, it remains a very gentle and supportive form of exercise – ideal for anyone concerned about back problems.

The Pilates system helps the back in several ways. It strengthens the muscles that support the back – not only those muscles within the back itself but also those that are crucial for core (and hence, back) strength, notably the abdominal muscles. It mobilizes the spine and releases stiff, rigid 'frozen' muscles and joints that lack flexibility. The exercises have a slow, relaxing rhythm, and help to release tension throughout the body, but particularly in the back, shoulders and neck. Finally, and perhaps most importantly, Pilates addresses the posture, concentrating on a strong, but relaxed, alignment of the spine which you learn to adopt not just when exercising but throughout the course of your everyday life.

With the help of Pilates technique, there is no need for the majority of those with back problems to suffer at all. This book is designed to help both those who have had back pain and those who wish to avoid it. As with any exercise system, check first with your doctor before you embark on it, particularly if you already have a back problem, then progress through the stages slowly and carefully for a stronger, healthier back.

Banish Back Pain the Pilates Way

How to Use This Book

There are many reasons that Pilates has become such a popular form of exercise. The main one, quite simply, is that it works. It is also very safe and gentle. To strengthen and safeguard your back, however, you must follow the steps in this book slowly and carefully, and you need to learn how to do the exercises properly. This means understanding the principles of the system and applying them so that you use your muscles in the most efficacious way.

As soon as you have recovered from back pain, I would strongly recommend that you have at least a few lessons with an experienced Pilates teacher before launching into the exercises in Part Three on your own. We all develop little quirks of posture and movement which, over time, can turn into bad habits – so sometimes you may think you are doing an exercise correctly when in fact you are using all the wrong muscles in an effort to simulate the photographs in the book. Because Pilates is such a precise science, you need to become very aware of how your body works and how to use it in the best possible way. A good teacher will help you do this.

As with any exercise regime, and particularly if you have already had back problems or any other concerns whatsoever about your health, you should consult your doctor before you begin. If you do have back problems, work thoroughly through the first levels before going on to anything more complex or difficult. And, if ever you feel any strain or pain in your back, or if your abdominal muscles start to bulge or quiver during an exercise, always stop immediately. These are indications that your muscles are not yet strong enough for what you are trying to do, so strengthen with exercises you can do without straining and come back to the harder ones when you're ready.

The book is divided into three main sections. Part One explains Pilates technique and how the exercises can help you. In Part Two there are exercises designed to mobilize your body very gently after you have had back pain, together with other methods to help you achieve short-term relief. In Part Three there are a series of progressively more difficult exercises to strengthen and mobilize your back and supporting muscles, increase flexibility and reduce tension and vulnerability to injury and pain. Because in Pilates you use your muscles in a very precise and controlled manner, you do not necessarily need to attempt the most difficult exercises. Providing you do the simpler exercises thoroughly and regularly, you will still improve the health of your back and give it protection for the future. The more difficult exercises will give you added strength, but if they are too much of a strain for your abdominal muscles, that strain will be transferred to your back – with the inevitable consequences of back pain or strain. So, just take it gently and work through each exercise fluently and accurately, only moving on to the next if your back feels really strong. Part Four then outlines some other manipulative techniques that can be used alongside Pilates.

Finally, from a general fitness point of view, there are some things that Pilates does not do. It is not an aerobic technique, so you will need to do some other form of exercise that raises your heart rate for 20 minutes three times each week. This also helps if you want to lose weight.

As I explain in more detail later, Pilates is a technique in which you need to concentrate, so it is worth creating an environment where it is possible for you to do so. Pick a time of day that suits you and when you are unlikely to be disturbed. Wear something comfortable that you can move easily in and that doesn't restrict your movements in any way. It is a good idea to get a yoga mat, especially for exercises where you are lying on your back, as working directly on the floor – even a carpet – will not give you as much support. The only other items you might need are towels, cushions, a long scarf or belt and a tennis ball. If it helps, you can exercise to music; this can help some people attain the rhythmic quality that is central to the technique. However, make sure the music is quiet and slow so that it establishes the right pace – slower is always better in Pilates technique. Finally, if you can, exercise in front of a mirror so you can check your postural alignment, which is of the utmost importance for your back.

Part One

1

What Is Pilates?

About 100 years ago the Pilates method originated near Düsseldorf in Germany when a frail youngster named Joseph Pilates took up body-building in an effort to increase his strength. At the time he was generally weak and sickly, and thought to be prone to tuberculosis, but the programme he devised was so successful that by the time he was 14, he was posing as a model for anatomical drawings.

He then went on to become an avid sportsman – diver, boxer, gymnast, skier, and even working as a circus performer. He left Germany in 1912, moving to England where, at the outbreak of the First World War he was interned. Pilates used this enforced leisure to develop his method of attaining peak physical fitness. He christened his system 'muscle contrology'. His aim was to bring about complete co-ordination of body, mind and spirit, by working with – not on or against – the body's muscles.

Pilates returned to Germany briefly after the war, and then moved to New York where his method was an instant success, particularly with dancers such as George Balanchine and Martha Graham. Until relatively recently it remained something of a secret among dancers, until sportspeople, actors and the general public discovered it. Its popularity has grown and grown over the past few years.

The Original Pilates Method

Pilates' early work centred primarily on aiding the rehabilitation of ill or injured people. During his internment Pilates worked as a nurse, experimenting with springs attached to hospital beds so that patients could work on toning their muscles even before they could get up and about. Springs, used as resistance, became the centrepiece of the method. Pilates designed a machine he called the 'universal reformer', a sliding horizontal bed which can be used with up to four springs, according to the particular exercise and the strength of the individual. On this machine, pliés and other exercises can be performed, without putting any stress on the joints (thus making them very beneficial for those with injuries or other joint problems) and against resistance (to work the muscles harder).

Pilates developed several other machines for his New York studio; these have been adapted and used around the world ever since. The principles of the Pilates method have also been adapted for use without machines, in a system which has become particularly popular. It is this version of Pilates that is used in this book.

2

The Pilates Principles

Although the Pilates method has changed significantly over the years, its underlying principles remain the same. In Pilates, every movement is carefully controlled for maximum effect. This requires concentration. For each and every exercise, there are questions you need to ask yourself. Is your navel drawn towards your spine? Is your neck long and aligned with your spine? Is your heel in the correct position? Are you breathing correctly?

The placing and movement of each part of your body counts in the Pilates system, and your body works as an integrated system. The more you use your body correctly during the exercises, the more you will use it correctly in everything you do. Your posture improves and any tightness and tension – and, above all, back problems – arising from poor posture will fade away.

Concentrating in this way will not leave you mentally drained or exhausted. On the contrary, it is a profoundly relaxing method of exercise and its slow, rhythmic movements are a stress-relief in themselves, leaving most people feeling both energized and calm.

The Principles

It is important to understand the underlying theory behind the Pilates method before you attempt the exercises. There are five essential principles to bear in mind.

Concentration

As mentioned, concentration is fundamental, not only because it is important that every part of your body is moving or positioned correctly – a part of a synchronized whole – but also because when you concentrate on your body in this way, your mind is led away from concerns or anxieties in a way that is profoundly relaxing.

The Breath

The way you breathe is vitally important within the Pilates method – you should breathe deeply, rhythmically and to your full capacity. The other point to remember is *when* to breathe. In Pilates exercises, you breathe out with the effort. This is not the way most people breathe – in fact, it's the opposite – but it does help you to relax into a movement. If you breathe in for the effort of an exercise, you will automatically tense up. This method of breathing is particularly important when using Pilates to help ease back problems, so that you avoid combining the effort of movement with the tension of inhaling.

The Girdle of Strength

Joseph Pilates used the term 'the girdle of strength'. The girdle incorporates three main areas – the back, the abdomen and the buttocks. If the muscles in this 'girdle' are weak, any weakness in your back is exacerbated, and your back becomes much more vulnerable to injury and strain.

The upper back in particular can be a major seat of tension, but when you learn to move your arms correctly (from the middle of your back rather than your shoulders), this tension, together with bunched muscles and stiffness, will disappear.

Nearly every exercise in this book begins by drawing the navel gently towards the spine. This strengthens the abdominal muscles – strong abdominal muscles are absolutely key to protecting and strengthening your back.

The third element in this girdle of strength is the buttock muscles. By squeezing and engaging these during the exercises, you tone the buttock muscles and bring your body into perfect alignment, improving your posture and protecting your back from injury and strain.

Flowing Movements

Sudden, jerky movements can be dangerous for your back. In Pilates, one position flows as slowly and naturally as possible into the next. The movements are rhythmic and the pace is set by your own breathing. This warms your muscles and lengthens them. Slow movements also give you time to become aware of each part of your body so that you perform all the exercises with precision and in a co-ordinated way.

Relaxation

The relaxation and breathing exercises are important elements of the Pilates method. The stresses and strains of modern living can result in bunched-up, tense muscles which in turn lead to headaches, back strain and injuries. Make sure you incorporate these exercises, as they will help relieve tension, restore flagging energy levels and, just as crucially, induce a tranquil state of mind.

3

Protecting Your Back

The spine is not straight, as many people assume. It is composed of 24 separate vertebrae stacked one on top of the other in the shape of three natural curves. These more or less graduate downwards in size, from the smallest at the neck to larger ones at the base, where the last vertebra is attached to the sacrum to form the spine's final curve. The sacrum is a curved, wedge-shaped bone that fits between the two hip bones of the pelvis, the ring of bone that supports the spine. Below this is the coccyx – the remains of a prehistoric tail.

The spine fulfils a number of vital functions. It supports almost all of the weight of the head and body. Its articulation and its supporting muscles give it – and us – the strength and mobility to bend, tilt, twist and lift. Finally, it protects the spinal cord, and thus the central nervous system, which connects the brain to every other part of the body.

To understand the spine properly, it is best to look at each of its three main sections in turn. The top section is the cervical spine, consisting of the seven vertebrae of the neck. Below this are the 12 vertebrae that make up the middle back, or thoracic spine. The lower back is the lumbar spine, with five vertebrae, the lowest of which connects to the sacrum at the back of the pelvis.

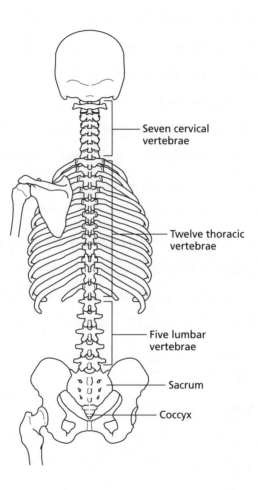

Seven cervical vertebrae

Twelve thoracic vertebrae

Five lumbar vertebrae

Sacrum

Coccyx

Each of these sections has a natural curve. The cervical spine has a lordotic, or concave, curve. The thoracic spine has a kyphotic, or convex, curve. The lumbar spine has another lordotic curve. At the sacrum, the coccyx forms a final kyphotic curve.

All three of the principal spinal sections can experience problems that result in varying kinds of 'bad back'. The most common of these is undoubtedly the lumbar (lower) spine, where low back pain can arise for a number of reasons. The central, thoracic, back can become rigid and inflexible, leading to stiffness and possible injury. The upper back, around the neck and shoulders, is one of the most common places to store tension, resulting not only in localized aches and pains but also headaches, migraines and other problems.

THE LUMBAR SPINE

The lowest section of the spine is the most vulnerable to strain and injury. This is not surprising when you consider that it bears so much of the weight of the upper body. The pressure of all this weight can compress the vertebrae together, increasing the likelihood of dysfunction in the lumbar area – and hence the possibility of low back pain and injury. This becomes even more likely if there are other factors: for example, if the abdominal muscles are weak, this puts great strain on the back during activities such as lifting. It used to be argued that if you had a bad back, exercise was the last thing you needed. Now, however, it is generally believed that while short-term rest for a maximum of two or three days is beneficial, most bad backs will benefit from gentle strengthening and mobilizing exercises.

To avoid lower back pain and injury, you should target the abdominal muscles and do exercises that stretch and release the compression of the lumbar spine. Good posture is vital to protect the lower back. The all-too-common exaggerated curve that produces a 'sway back' (usually accompanied by a bulging stomach) destabilizes the lumbar region and leaves it particularly vulnerable to weakness and pain.

THE THORACIC SPINE

Without proper exercise, the area of the middle back can become very stiff and rigid. In time, this can result in an exaggerated kyphotic curve, so that the chest caves in and the middle back becomes rounded. Such stiffness combined with poor posture causes the back to lose suppleness and resilience, again making injury more likely.

To address this type of problem, you should do exercises that increase flexibility, including gentle stretching, bending and twisting. Good posture is also very important to correct any exaggerated curves.

THE CERVICAL SPINE

The upper spine is particularly prone to tension from all sorts of causes – physical, mental and emotional. The more tension you store, the worse the muscular problems become. This can lead to shoulder and neck ache, as well as headache and migraine. Muscular tension also makes injury more likely – as in 'cricking' your neck. Common postural problems in this part of the back include rigid, hunched or rounded shoulders and the chin jutting too far forwards or pulled too far back – both of which distort the upper spine.

Exercises for this area include releasing the neck and shoulders from tension to make them more mobile and learning good postural placement. Relaxation techniques are also important.

The Vertebrae and Discs

Each of the three sections of the spine is composed of a series of vertebrae, arranged to form a column. All the vertebrae have a similar basic structure – though with variations throughout the length of the spine – consisting of two separate 'compartments'. The front compartment is round and weight-bearing. The back compartment, which contains the spinal cord, locks the vertebrae together and has 'wings' linked to the muscles, which make the vertebrae move.

The front compartment of each vertebra is interleaved with intervertebral discs. These discs are cushioning pads that act as shock-absorbers and stop the bones grinding against each other. The discs are composed of a tough, elastic outer wall housing a liquid, jelly-like centre, called the nucleus. The nucleus can be squashed down and change its shape under pressure, but when you lie down the pressure is taken off, water is drawn in and the nucleus swells up again. The result of this is that, after a night's sleep, first thing in the morning you are very slightly taller than you are at the end of the day! The nuclei of children's discs are nearly 90 per cent water, but this percentage decreases with age, shortening the spine as we grow older.

The discs have no blood supply of their own; they receive oxygen and nutrients as a side-effect of spinal movement – so the more you move, the healthier and plumper the discs will be. This may seem strange, as it is often a sudden movement that can 'put your back out'. However, when your back is both strong and flexible from regular exercise, movement is not a threat to it.

Everyone has heard of a slipped disc – for a long time regarded as the principal culprit when it came to bad backs. However, it is now generally acknowledged that discs don't slip, they burst – and this, in turn, means that they are permanently damaged and can't simply be put back into the right place. Fortunately, this is a much rarer event than 'slipped' discs were once thought to be.

The Muscles and Other Structures of the Back

The spine is kept upright by several groups of muscles. The strength of these muscles directly affects the well-being of your back. The spinal muscles themselves are, relatively speaking, quite small, and lie in two sets on either side of the spine (no muscles cross over the backbone) in a mirror image of each other. Layers criss-cross each other, the largest being the diagonal muscles of the top layer that run from the spine to the shoulders. Below these are long muscles extending from the pelvis up to the ribs, the vertebrae and the head. Deepest of all, there are small muscles that link the vertebrae together.

Just as important for spinal health, however, are the abdominal muscles. If the abdominal muscles are strong, they support the back. If not, the back takes more of the strain – during both exercise and everyday activities – than it should. The abdominal muscles are key in maintaining good posture and spinal alignment, as well as in a wide range of movements, such as twisting and bending. Strong abdominal muscles are vital to protect the back when you lift a heavy weight or do a sit-up.

The spine is also strengthened by a network of ligaments – fibrous bands of tissue – at each point where two bones form a joint. The ligaments control a joint's range of movement and connect the spine to the pelvis and the rib cage.

In the spaces between these elements is connective tissue, mostly comprising a protein substance called collagen. Collagen conveys nutrients from the bloodstream to the muscles and ligaments, and removes waste products from them for elimination.

Finally, the spinal cord lies within the spinal column, encased within the dural tube – three layers of tubular membrane. It links the brain to every part of the body via a network of nerves that branch out from the spinal cord.

4

What Can Go Wrong?

There are all sorts of different reasons why people experience back pain – just as there are many different kinds of back pain. Often it is difficult to locate precisely the source of the problem, and it is very likely that, as the discs, nerves, muscles and joints of the back are all inter-related, more than one part of your back is involved. It is not within the scope of this book to deal with specific medical problems in detail. However, here is a brief summary of some of the possible origins of back pain.

Injury and Accidents

An injury – whiplash after a car accident, for instance – is perhaps one of the easiest causes of back pain to pinpoint. Sporting injuries are very common, too, particularly in highly active or potentially dangerous sports such as skiing, riding or parachuting. Even injuries, however, are not always clear cut. If your back goes into spasm after lifting a heavy weight, it may be a result of cumulative back stress due to an underlying problem of weak muscles or poor posture. Often you don't even need to incur an obvious strain on the back – if there is a fundamental weakness your back may go into spasm even if you just cough or sneeze.

If after examination following an accident there seems to be no need for surgery or other medical treatment, an initial period of rest is usually recommended (see page 40). This may be accompanied by painkillers and hot and cold treatments (see page 42) and followed by gentle exercise designed to bring mobility back to the injured area. Very often, the pain itself is caused by muscles going into spasm as a result of the shock of the accident or injury, in an involuntary response aimed at protecting the spine from further trauma. Muscle spasm slows down the healing process, however, so it is vital to release this as soon as possible (see page 42).

Scoliosis

This is a condition in which the spine is bent to one side, giving it (when viewed from the back) an 'S' shape. It may occur as a result of injury, bone disease, poor posture or having one leg shorter than the other. It is quite a common condition, at least to a small degree, and can put extra stress on the back. This, in turn, may increase the risk of further pain and injury.

Arthritis

Arthritis is a general term covering two major ailments. Osteoarthritis is a degenerative condition that affects the spine as well as other bones of the body. It can occur as a result of general wear and tear on the spine, especially if the discs between the vertebrae shrink so that the vertebrae themselves get closer together and perhaps rubs against each other. Osteoarthritis occurs mostly as we get older and, although some people do experience symptoms, others may remain unaware that they have the condition.

Rheumatoid arthritis less commonly affects the back than the limbs, hands and other parts of the body. When it is found in the spine, it usually affects the neck and lumbar areas.

If you have arthritis, you should consult your doctor before you start any of the exercises in this book.

Osteoporosis

Although it can occur in men and in younger women, osteoporosis most often affects post-menopausal women. Its common name is 'brittle bone disease' and it gives rise to the demineralization of the bones – especially the loss of calcium – causing the spine, in particular, to degenerate. At its worst, this can result in the rounded back known as 'dowager's hump' and can cause the spine to shrink, resulting in loss of height. Osteoporosis also affects other bones and is a direct cause of hip fracture – the bones becoming more brittle and therefore more easy to break – and the increasing need of hip replacements for the elderly.

Diet is very important in the fight against osteoporosis. Calcium and vitamin D are an essential part of a healthy diet, both found in milk, butter and eggs. Vitamin D is also formed directly in the skin by exposure to sunlight. If you have osteoporosis, consult your doctor before trying the exercises in this book.

Spondylitis

Spondylitis or Ankylosing spondylitis is a condition in which the joints of the back lose their mobility and the spine can become completely rigid. The rigidity causes the back to become rounded rather than straight, so that a stoop develops – a kyphotic curve where there should be a lordotic one. It affects men more than women and it is rare nowadays to see a severe case. However, mild cases are still common. Symptoms of low back stiffness and pain occur in the morning. These wear off during the day, with movement, though they may return after prolonged sitting. Treatment entails correcting your posture and taking physiotherapy and exercise. Check with your doctor before starting the exercises in this book if you have or suspect you have spondylitis.

Spondylolisthesis

Spondylolisthesis means 'slipping vertebrae'. It is a condition where one vertebra slips forward out of alignment with the vertebra below it. It is most common in the lumbar spine and this, in turn, affects the alignment of the spine above the slippage. The problem may be hereditary or caused by injury or accident. The less common, backward slippage is called retrolisthesis.

Weight and Height

Being overweight is a serious risk factor for both causing and aggravating back problems. The effect of obesity is to increase the strain on the back during all day-to-day movements – such as walking, getting up from a chair, lifting or bending. It is, quite simply, harder for the back to do any of these simple tasks because it is labouring under an extra weight all the time. If you are overweight and suffer from back problems, one of your first priorities should be to try to lose some weight.

Very tall people are also more likely to develop back problems, often caused by bending and lifting. If you are tall, therefore, it is even more important to correct your posture and take particular care when bending forward or lifting heavy objects.

Pregnancy

Pregnancy puts an extra strain on the back because, with the increasing weight of the baby, your posture tends to change to carry the extra load. Typically, this results in overarching the lower back, leading to back pain. During the later stages of pregnancy, the ligaments soften and become looser so that the pelvis can accommodate the baby's delivery. This can result in straining or overstretching; particular care is needed, especially during exercise. Sacro-iliac pain – in the joints that connect the sacrum or tail bone to the pelvis – is very common during pregnancy. The ligaments return to normal in the first few months after the birth but you should always consult your doctor if you are pregnant or if you have recently had a baby before you start any exercise routine. For more detailed information on Pilates exercises that are suitable during pregnancy, see my earlier book, *Pilates for Pregnancy*.

Referred Pain

One rather confusing element in back pain is referred pain. The confusion arises from the fact that, though the cause of the pain originates in the back, the pain itself is felt elsewhere. Most commonly, pain is felt in the back of the thigh due to a trapped sciatic nerve in the spine. Referred pain also works the other way round – pain originating in another part of the body can be felt in the back. These typically include peptic ulcers and period pain.

Non-specific Back Pain

It is often impossible to pinpoint a specific illness or event that is the root cause of back pain. In these cases, it is almost certainly down to lifestyle. Because most of us these days live quite sedentary lives, our backs are not used as they should be. Slouching is widespread from childhood onwards, and poor posture puts a great strain on the back, weakening the supporting muscles and leading to an increased likelihood of back injury.

Sedentary work means more and more people spend hours every day in a fixed position – usually with poor back support and equally poor posture. Lack of exercise leads to weak muscles in the back and, more importantly, in the abdomen, putting yet more stress on the spine. All of these factors combine to decrease mobility in the spine, making it more rigid and vulnerable to strain.

Finally, there is stress. It is now widely accepted that mental or emotional stress often transforms itself into muscle tension. And it does seem that the back is one of the main places where tension is stored. The neck and shoulders – as many people know to their cost – are prime examples. As tension invades this area, you may hear worrying clicks if you try to rotate your shoulders, and it is often one mass of knotty tension, as most masseurs can attest. Tension headaches are another common result. Muscle spasm due to unexpressed tension and worries can also be located in other parts of the back – for example, some people believe it can result in a rigid thoracic (middle) or lumbar (lower) spine.

5

How Pilates
Can Help

Pilates exercises can help to protect your back against injury and pain in several important ways. Many of the most common back problems are due to the weakness of the muscles that support the back, and to poor posture. Pilates is designed to strengthen these muscles, while simultaneously correcting your posture. The exercises are gentle and effect a gradual but safe improvement so you can work towards a stronger back without fear of pain or injury.

Pilates also works to increase flexibility – and this is particularly important for spinal health. The exercises aim to reduce stored tension in the muscles and to make the back (and, in fact, all the joints) more mobile. This is supported by another key area in Pilates technique – relaxation. The exercises that follow in the book focus on four key areas:

- *The neck and shoulders* This area suffers from tension, stiffness and lack of mobility. The Pilates exercises open up the area, making it freer and looser, reducing stored muscular tension and improving posture, notably the position of the head and rounded shoulders.

- *Thoracic back* The middle back is often the stiffest part of the back, and this rigidity can cause it not only to be more vulnerable to strain and pain, but severely restrict breathing and undermine your posture.

- *Lower back* This is the most common place for back pain. It is the part of the spine that is put under most pressure, as it supports the whole of the back and is particularly undermined by poor posture, especially over-arching in small of back. Lack of flexibility can also make it vulnerable to injury.

- *Abdominal muscles* Though not part of the back itself, the abdominal muscles are crucial to its health. They must be strong and well toned to support the posture and to maintain the back's strength and flexibility.

Part Two

6

Gently Mobilizing Your Back

Prevention is always better than cure, especially for the misery of a bad back. But if you already have acute (sudden, severe) back pain, there are several steps you can take to relieve it before you go on to strengthen your back and avoid future recurrences. If you have chronic (on-going) back pain, you will not need bed rest, but check out possibilities for pain relief, then go straight to the exercises beginning on page 44.

Bed Rest

For a long time, long-term bed rest was deemed to be the answer for acute bad backs. Nowadays, however, this advice has changed and mobility is seen as vital to a swifter, more complete recovery. If you stay in bed too long, you stiffen up and movement becomes even more difficult, so the sooner you begin to do some gentle exercises designed to bring muscle release and relaxation to the afflicted area, the better it will be.

Having said this, very short-term bed rest can be beneficial. If you are in agony after a sudden sprain or injury, the only thing you can do is to rest and, in fact, this will in most cases gradually help you to relax and ease the pain. Because your muscles go into a spasm in a reflex action designed to protect the injured area – and prevent you from doing it any more harm – until these muscles relax, there is little you can do.

It is important, though, to get the most benefit from bed rest that you can. This will depend upon the way you lie down. Don't be tempted to lie face-down – this will only cause you to arch your lumbar spine. It is best to lie either on your back or on your side. If you are lying on your back, have just one pillow under your head. If you have more, your back will tend to slump into an unsupported curve. Pillows are put to better use under your knees. This position releases the lower back and, in some cases, relieves a lot of pain immediately. Depending on what feels most comfortable, you can just put one pillow so that your knees are slightly bent, or a whole heap of them so that your knees form a right angle, with your calves supported on the pillows. Lying with your knees supported in this way puts your back in correct alignment and gently stretches out your back muscles.

If you prefer, you can reproduce this position by lying on the floor with your feet and lower legs on a chair. However, this should only be done for a short period, as bed rest – and most beds are usually quite supportive enough, so the floor or a board beneath the mattress is not generally required – yields the most benefits when you are lying still for a prolonged length of time doing nothing at all. If you have a particularly soft mattress that you feel is not giving you sufficient support, put one or two thick blankets or quilts on the floor and lie on top. Remember, though, that one of the benefits of being in bed is that you are warm – and this helps to relax your muscles – so keep warm.

If you find lying on your back too uncomfortable, try lying on your side. Bend your knees and put a pillow between them to support your upper leg and to prevent twisting your spine. If the pain is in your neck, you may benefit from a special neck pillow – it supports your neck and sides of your head. As the pain starts to abate, try some of the gentlest exercises in the next section beginning on page 44.

Pain Relief

As your immediate aim is to release your muscles from spasm – and stop the pain! – you will probably need to use some kind of pain relief for an acute bad back. The best tactic is to use a painkiller that offers you powerful relief for a short time so that, in the absence of pain, the muscles can relax. Remember that most of these kinds of medications should be taken with food.

In some cases, your doctor may prescribe muscle relaxants. These are often tranquillizers under another name and, again, should be taken for only a short time as some types can become addictive.

If you suffer from a chronic bad back, painkillers are not an option, given the long-term toxic build-up that would result. TENS (Transcutaneous Electric Nerve Stimulation) is an electrical therapy that transmits an electrical current to the painful area, thus breaking the cycle of pain and muscle spasm. Many people find acupuncture is very helpful in back-pain relief, while massage is not only beneficial for the pain, it is a very uplifting and relaxing therapy (see page 190) which, as well as releasing specific knots of muscle, also relieves generally the tension that accompanies back pain.

Applying either extreme heat or extreme cold to the source of pain can also be very effective. As a general rule of thumb, cold applications are used for acute pain immediately after injury and for a day or two beyond. Hot applications are best for chronic back pain.

If you are applying an ice pack, you can use whatever you have to hand in the first instance – a bag of frozen peas, for instance. If you are going to be using this treatment regularly you can use a hot water bottle filled with ice cubes, or a freezer ice pack, though you must wrap it in a towel first, as direct contact with the skin can cause ice burns. Apply the pack to the source of pain for up to 20 minutes every hour.

The best heat pack is just a hot water bottle – and again this should be wrapped in a towel. Place on the source of pain for up to half an hour, repeating every two hours. A hot bath can also help to relax muscle spasm – but make sure you have someone to help you out of the bath or, alternatively, try a hot shower.

Gentle Exercises for Back Pain

The exercises here are, strictly speaking, more movements than exercises proper, designed to keep the body moving – however slightly – when you are suffering from back pain, even from the time of bed rest. Although rest can be very beneficial immediately after a back problem has begun, it is generally accepted nowadays that the rest should not be prolonged or, far from relieving the problem, you will stiffen up and re-mobilizing will be harder than ever. Muscles can lose their strength remarkably quickly – it is estimated that after just 10 days of bed rest, the strength of your thigh muscles can diminish by up to a third.

Movement also stimulates the circulation, bringing oxygen and nutrients to the area and carrying away toxins. As back pain is part of a vicious circle of tension, relaxation and breathing techniques can be immensely helpful, too.

If at any time an exercise causes you pain, stop immediately.

FIRST EXERCISES

All of the following exercises are designed to bring mobility back and to relax muscle spasm. They can be done while you are still in bed. For maximum benefit, intersperse movement with breathing or relaxation techniques.

For all of these exercises, lie on your bed without a pillow – though you can use one during the breathing or relaxation techniques if you find this more comfortable. As the pain eases and you become more mobile, you can do these exercises on the floor, using a yoga mat or something similar to protect your spine. Repeat those you can do without pain up to five times a day – the more mobile your back becomes, the more quickly it is likely to be better.

Toe-wriggling

It really is as simple as it sounds. Lying flat in bed or with your knees slightly raised, wriggle your toes, scrunching and stretching them for up to a minute. Then stretch them out as far as they will go, holding the stretch while you take five long, slow breaths.

Ankle circles

Lying flat in bed, slowly bend and stretch your feet from the ankles up to 5 times. Then, starting with your feet flexed back and your toes pointing towards the ceiling, slowly circle them so your toes point away from each other. Continue the circle so that your toes stretch away from you, then inwards back to the starting position, so your toes are again pointing towards the ceiling. Do this up to 5 times.

Breathing

Lying with your knees supported by a pillow, place your hands on your abdomen with your fingers just touching. Take a long, slow breath, feeling the breath travel through your lungs and down towards your abdomen so that it fills with air and your fingers part. Slowly exhale so that your fingers meet up again. Repeat up to 10 times, concentrating as much as you can on the breath as it travels through your body.

Knee to Chest

1. Lying in bed, raise your knees so that your feet are flat on the mattress. Let your lower spine relax as much as possible, reducing the curve in the small of your back.

2. Breathe in and, as you breathe out, draw your navel towards your spine and slowly raise one knee towards your chest. If this is painful, or becomes painful as you reach a certain point, stop. If you can, hold your leg below your knee and gently draw it closer to your chest and hold it there for a few moments. Don't tense your upper body, particularly your shoulders, neck and face.

3. Breathe in and, as you breathe out, return your leg to the starting position and repeat with the other leg. Alternate up to 5 times on each leg, resting and breathing deeply between each movement and taking care to keep your navel drawn in and your lower back stretched out on each movement.

Knee to Chest with a Pelvic Tilt

This exercise builds on the last one so do not try it unless you can do the previous one without pain. Again, move slowly and take deep breaths between each movement.

1. Lie on your back with your knees raised, as in the previous exercise. Breathe in and, as you breathe out, draw your navel to your spine, slightly curling up your pelvis and tightening your buttock muscles.

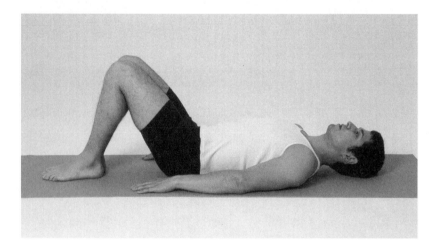

2. Holding this position, draw your knee to your chest and hold for a few moments. Breathe in and, as you breathe out, return to the starting position, releasing your buttock muscles.

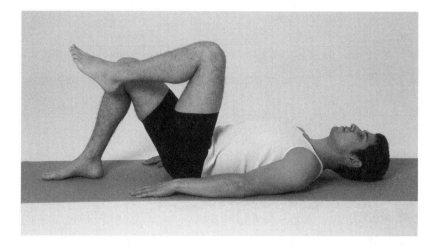

3. Alternate up to 5 times on each leg, taking long, deep breaths between each movement.

Head Raises

This exercise entails only a small movement but it should be done very slowly. If there is any pain, stop immediately.

1. Lie on your back with your knees raised and your feet flat on the bed. Check that there is no tension in your upper body, particularly in your shoulders or neck. Take a few long, deep breaths and try to relax further. Place your hands, fingers just touching, on your abdomen.

2. Breathe in and, as you breathe out, draw your navel towards your spine and make a small pelvic tilt as you raise your head to look down towards your knees. This can be only a very small movement – there is no need to raise your head off the bed if you feel any pain. If there is no pain, however, try to lift your head up slowly, then down again slowly. If your neck or shoulders tense up, you are lifting up too far.

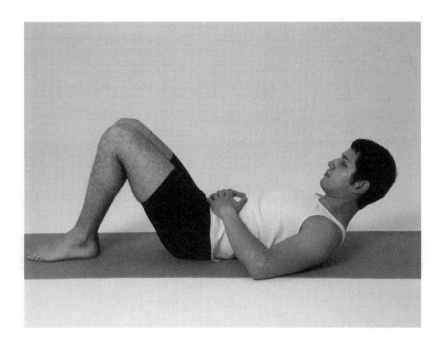

3. Repeat up to 5 times, resting between movements as necessary.

Leg Extensions

This exercise helps to bring awareness of pelvic stability and stretches out your back. Don't force your leg further than it can comfortably go; if you feel any pain, stop immediately.

1. Lie on your back with your knees raised and your feet flat on the floor or mattress.

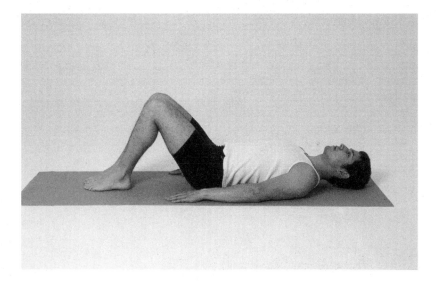

2. Take a long, slow breath in and, as you breathe out, start to slide your left foot away from you.

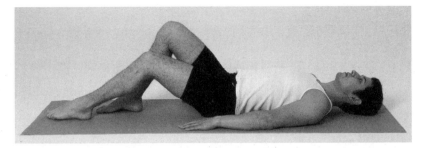

3. Take it as far as you can – the aim is to have your leg on the floor or bed. If you can get your leg flat, then flex your foot so that your toes point up towards the ceiling. If you can't take the stretch so far, don't worry – just go as far as you can.

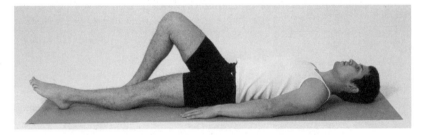

4. Hold the stretch for a moment, taking a long, slow breath in and out. Then, on the next out-breath, slide your foot up to its starting point and repeat with the other leg.

5. Repeat very slowly, alternating legs, up to 5 times on each side. If you can do this comfortably and without changing the position of your pelvis, you can try it with both legs together.

Gently Mobilizing Your Back   **53**

Twist

This exercise gives your back a diagonal stretch and it is very useful for relaxing muscle spasm – providing it has already relaxed to some degree. If it hasn't, this may hurt and you should leave this exercise for later.

1. Lie on your back with your knees raised, your feet flat on the floor or mattress. Place your arms in a wide 'V' just below shoulder height and check there is no tension in your shoulders or neck. Place a thin cushion between your knees.

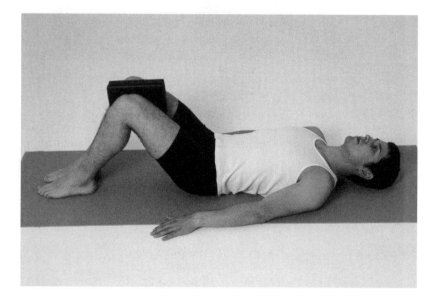

2. Breathe in and, as you breathe out, lower your knees to the left, keeping the cushion in place (you will need to grip with your knees to do this) and keeping as much of your spine as possible in contact with the floor or mattress. You should feel a pleasant stretch across your lower back, abdomen and thighs. Only go as far as you can in comfort, though. Hold the stretch while you take three long, slow breaths and relax into the position. If holding your knees in this position is difficult for you, you may find it helpful to rest them against the wall or a pile of cushions.

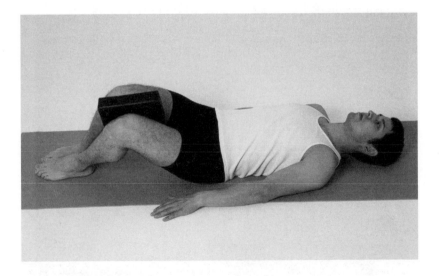

3. Return to the starting position and then repeat, taking your knees to the right.

RELAXATION

After or between exercises, it is important for you to relax. Relaxation will help both to release the muscle spasm and to make you feel more calm and positive about overcoming the problem. This sequence should take between 10 and 15 minutes – it depends on your own timing. Don't be tempted to rush it – this is a very valuable part of your routine.

The relaxation takes place in what is known in yoga as the Corpse Pose. If you are still in bed, you will obviously do your relaxation there. However, as your back starts to feel better, it is preferable to do your relaxation on a yoga mat on the floor.

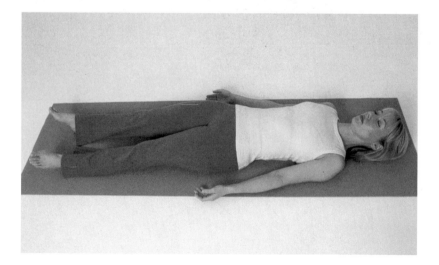

Many people find it helpful to record the following instructions on tape and play it while they do the relaxation. If you do this, ensure you speak very slowly, repeating each instruction several times.

During the relaxation, your body temperature will drop so, if you are not in bed, cover yourself with a blanket or put on an extra layer of clothing, especially socks, as your feet can get cold.

1. Lie down with your spine long and your arms close to your sides, palms uppermost. It may seem more natural to face the palms down, but when they are facing up your upper back and shoulders are lowered and so less likely to be tensed. Close your eyes and give yourself a few moments in which to become aware of the weight of your whole body, softening and relaxing. If you can, roll your head gently from side to side to check there is no tension in your neck.

2. Starting at your toes, begin to feel the relaxation spreading through your body, moving upwards like a wave. Spend time on each tiny part, putting all your concentration into each area of your body in turn – first your toes, then your feet and ankles.

3. Feel the wave spreading up into your legs, through your shins and calves, your knees and into your thighs. Let your legs roll outwards from your hips. Let your hips and buttocks go – there is often a surprising amount of tension stored here.

4. Your whole body is now softer. The effect now reaches your abdomen, which drops down further against your back, relaxing your lower spine.

5. Your stomach, waist and ribs all expand and soften. Your breathing is now probably quite light. As the softening, relaxing wave flows through your torso and into your back, they fall deeper into the mattress or floor. The relaxation comes up into your shoulders and neck and out along your arms to the very ends of your fingers. The back of your neck is almost touching the floor, your scalp softens, almost loose against your skull, and your whole face – jaw, chin, throat and cheeks – feel like they're melting away. Your lips part and your tongue rests gently behind your lower teeth. Your eyes sink softly back into your head and your temples and forehead smooth out.

6. Your whole body is at rest. Enjoy this sensation, be aware of it. As thoughts come into your mind, watch them and see them float away

like clouds in a summer sky. Any doubts or worries can float away in the same manner as physical tension leaves your body. Stay in this place for 3-5 minutes. Now see the sun in your sky and feel its life-giving light and warmth. Feel the air around you and, as you take a deep breath in, feel that you are drinking in from the sun's vast source of energy, making you calmer and stronger.

7. Now begin to deepen the breath, letting your ribs expand and your lungs fill. After three breaths, begin to feel your toes and fingers coming to life. Wriggle them. Still with your eyes closed, lift your arms above your head and stretch your arms and legs away from each other. When you are ready, open your eyes.

How to Protect Your Back in Everyday Movements

As your back starts to improve, you will want to return to normal life as much as possible. This is the time to begin the exercises in Part Three, and also to find ways to protect your back from strain and injury during everyday activities. The key to this is posture. Pilates technique is designed to correct your posture, bringing your spine into proper alignment and thus making it less vulnerable. This proper alignment is not just for use during exercise, though, so this section helps you to become more generally aware of your posture and how you can improve it. You can also protect your back during everyday movements – such as lifting, sitting, getting out of bed and driving – and there is advice on how to perform these activities safely.

POSTURE

Posture may seem an old-fashioned word, but it is of the utmost importance to all of us – and especially those who are vulnerable to back pain or strain. By ensuring that your posture is good all the time – not just when you are exercising – every movement you make becomes a way of protecting your spine and toning and strengthening your body.

Many people have spines that end up in an exaggerated S shape and, when this happens, pains and strains are inevitable. What you should be aiming at, instead, is a long but relaxed stance. It is a good idea to check your posture not only before you start each exercise session but also regularly in your everyday life. Stand in front of a mirror, preferably with another one set up to give you a side view, too. Here are the main points to look out for.

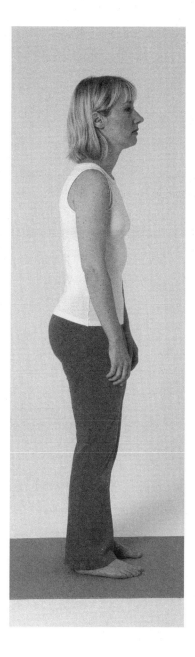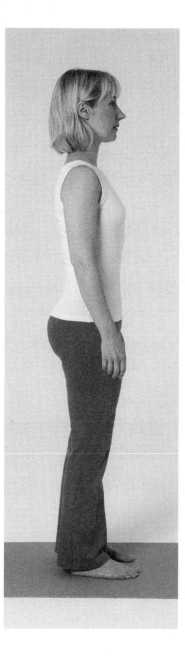

Gently Mobilizing Your Back

Head and Neck

Your head should sit relaxed and balanced at the top of your spine with your neck long and in line with your spine. If you tip your chin up or jut it out, you will pull your neck out of alignment with your spine and this distortion will have serious consequences for your posture, creating tension in several muscle groups and, quite possibly, back pain, strain or headaches. Your chin should be tipped very slightly down to lengthen the back of your neck and you should feel as if the top of your head is attached to a piece of string pulling you up and lengthening you out.

Shoulders and Arms

Your shoulders and upper back often hold a great deal of the body's tension, much of it due to incorrect posture. All arm movements should originate in the muscles of your middle back, beneath your shoulder blades, and the shoulders themselves should not lift up just because your arms do. Lift your shoulders up to your ears and just let them drop down into a relaxed position – this is where they should be all of the time. Your arms should hang comfortably by your sides, without tension. Looking straight at the mirror, check that your shoulders are at an even height – sometimes one is tensed and held higher than the other, especially if you always carry a bag on the same side. Turn sideways to the mirror and check that your shoulders are neither pulled back (which distorts your neck) or slouched forwards.

Back and Stomach

Stand sideways to the mirror to check your back. Let your spine lengthen out, your tailbone dropping towards the floor. Draw your navel gently towards your spine so that you do not overarch in the small of your back and your bottom does not stick out. Using these muscles protects your back from strain and is part of the Pilates 'girdle of strength'.

Buttocks

When your navel and back are in the correct placement, your pelvis will tilt very slightly upwards. If you gently squeeze the lowest muscles in your buttocks, this will help you maintain the correct alignment.

Legs and Feet

Your feet should be hip-width apart, toes facing forwards, not turned out. Your legs should feel long and pulled up without overextending your knee, pushing it too far back. Feel the weight evenly distributed between both feet.

POSTURAL EXERCISES

The following three exercises are designed to help you become more aware of your posture and to correct it by feeling how you should be placing your spine – and the rest of your body. Do these exercises regularly, both as a spot-check on your posture and as a warm-up for the exercises in Part Three.

Roll Down Against Wall

This exercise mobilizes and places your spine in its correct alignment. The more slowly you do this exercise, the better. Try to feel each vertebra as you draw it away or place it against the wall. You will find it is your abdominal muscles that do the work of controlling your body's alignment – but you should also check that there is no tension anywhere (particularly in your neck, shoulders or back).

1. Stand 12–18 inches away from a wall with your knees slightly bent and your feet hip-width apart, toes facing forwards. Measure out the entire length of your spine against the wall (no gaps), with your head

held high on a long neck and your shoulders relaxed. Let your arms hang comfortably at your sides.

2. Breathe in and, as you breathe out, draw your navel gently towards your spine and drop your chin to your chest, feeling the stretch all the way through your neck and upper back. As you begin to mobilize your spine, your arms will move naturally – just let them hang, don't try to place them.

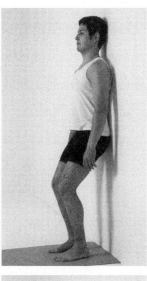

3. Let the curve deepen so your back peels away from the wall in a long, relaxed curve, your head and arms hanging until only your buttocks are touching the wall. Breathe naturally for a few moments as your body hangs upside down and releases into the stretch.

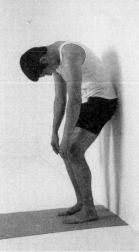

Gently Mobilizing Your Back

4. On the next out-breath, check that your navel is still drawn towards your spine and rotate from your pelvis to bring yourself back to a standing position, feeling your back touch the wall vertebra by vertebra. As your back unrolls, feel your shoulders drop down naturally. Let your head come in line with your spine, last of all. Check that your back is long, your neck and shoulders are relaxed and your 'girdle of strength' is working. Repeat this exercise 3 times.

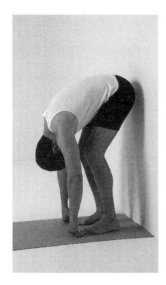

Slide Down Wall

This is another postural exercise. It lengthens the spine, teaches correct alignment and works the thigh muscles.

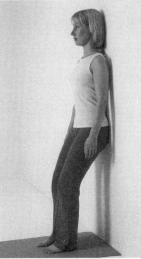

1. Stand as you did in the previous exercise and measure out the length of your spine against the wall, with your head held high on a long neck and your shoulders relaxed. Let your arms hang comfortably at your sides.

2. Breathe in and, as you breathe out, draw your navel gently to your spine and bend your knees more deeply so that your back starts to slide down the wall. Take care not to go any further than your thighs are able to support your weight without lifting your heels off the floor or letting any part of your back come away from the wall.

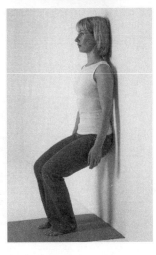

3. Breathe in and slide back up. Repeat up to 5 times.

Gently Mobilizing Your Back

Finding Neutral

This exercise is designed to develop awareness of where your spine and abdominal muscles should be placed, not just when you are exercising but also in your everyday life. This placement is vital to the accurate performance of the exercises that follow in Part Three.

1. Lie on your back with your knees bent and your feet flat on the floor, parallel (toes facing straight ahead) and in line with your hips. You can put a thin cushion under your head if it makes you more comfortable. Your arms should be relaxed by your sides with no tension in your shoulders – if you prefer to feel the extent of the movement more strongly, place your hands on your abdomen. You will find there is a natural curve in your back and – the extent varies from individual to individual – some of your spine will not be in contact with the floor.

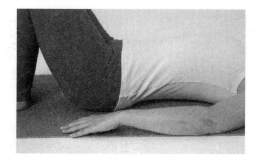

2. Now, curl your buttocks up and feel your spine flatten out along the floor. This is a pelvic tilt and, while it is needed in some exercises, in others it would distort the correct working of the muscles.

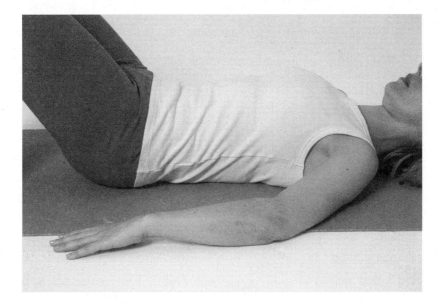

3. Now, replace your buttocks on the floor, curving in the opposite direction so that your back hollows out and widens the gap between your spine and the floor. Your abdomen will bulge out. This is a position you should never use regularly – though it is a common postural problem – as in this position you cannot work your abdominal muscles and you can put a potentially dangerous strain on your back.

4. Return to the first position and feel your spine long and relaxed with a slight arch around the small of your back. Draw your abdominal muscles gently towards your spine, but without distorting it or moving your pelvis, so they are held lightly but firmly. This is your neutral position. Unless the exercise you are doing entails a pelvic tilt, this is the placement in which you will perform most of the movements.

Everyday Movements

Most back problems come not as a result of an unavoidable injury but because of the way we perform everyday movements. The strain is cumulative – one day your back just 'goes' when you are performing an action you have done thousands of times before. To minimize this strain, you may need to learn some simple techniques for these day-to-day movements.

LIFTING

This is one of the most risky movements – it is very easy to put an unbearable strain on your back, particularly if you are lifting a heavy weight. If you know your back is vulnerable, always think carefully before you lift. If the weight looks as if it will be too much, don't put your back at risk. And if you are going to lift something, follow these guidelines to minimize risk and so that your legs take most of the strain instead of your back:

- Whenever possible – carrying shopping, for instance – divide the load into two equal parts, one for each hand.
- Bend your knees before you lift, with one foot in front of the other for a firm base – the front foot flat on the floor, the back foot raised onto the ball.
- Keep your back as straight as possible.
- As you lift, straighten your legs, using the thigh muscles to come up slowly.
- Breathe in to prepare, and then draw your navel to your spine and lift on the out-breath.

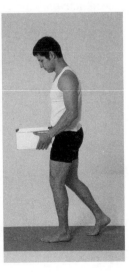

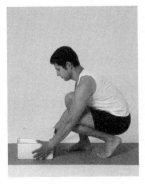
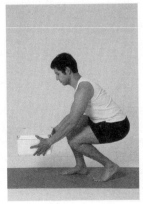

SITTING

If you spend most of your working life sitting at a desk, it is very important that you have a chair with good support for your back. Some people like kneeling chairs where much of your weight rests on your knees and, though this chair has no back, your spine is automatically placed in alignment. Otherwise, choose a chair that has a firm seat at the right height for you to place your feet flat on the floor with your knees at right angles. The most important place for the back to be supported is in the lumbar spine. Other points to bear in mind when sitting:

- Do not cross your legs at the feet or ankles, but keep your feet flat on the floor.
- Don't slump – keep your back as straight as possible.
- Get up from the chair by moving to the edge of the seat, putting one foot in front of the other and bending at the hips, not by arching your lower back.
- Arrange your work area to avoid twisting movements.
- Don't wedge the phone between your shoulder and ear.
- As often as possible, stand up and walk around or do some stretching

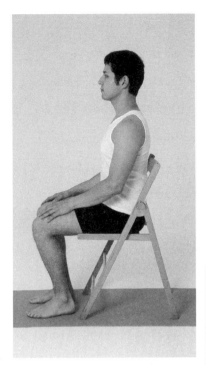

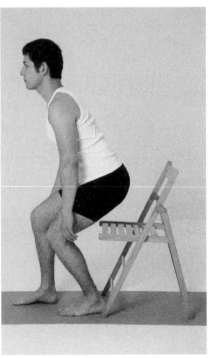

Gently Mobilizing Your Back 73

LYING DOWN

As has already been said, lying face-down on your bed increases the arch in your lower spine, so it is better to lie on your back or side. Your mattress does not need to be hard, but it should be firm. Feather pillows (rather than foam) offer more support to your neck.

GETTING OUT OF BED

When you get out of bed in the morning or get up from the floor after exercising, roll on to your side first. Swing your legs off the bed or, if getting up from the floor, push yourself up on your hands and come to a kneeling position first.

DRIVING

The guidelines for driving are similar to those for sitting at your desk.

- Keep your back as straight as possible.
- Keep your knees in line with your buttocks.
- Have your arms bent – don't stretch out for the steering wheel.
- Stop and walk about frequently, if only for a few minutes.

Part Three

7

Exercises to Strengthen and Support Your Back

A strong, flexible back is pain free. This section of the book gives you a step-by-step guide to strengthening your back and its supporting muscles, including, most importantly, the abdominal and leg muscles. There are also exercises for improving posture, increasing flexibility, removing muscle tension and achieving relaxation.

It is very important to go at your own pace, particularly if you have already suffered from back pain. Above all, if at any time you feel pain, stop immediately.

Many of the exercises that follow require strength in the abdominal muscles. If those muscles are not yet strong enough, it is your back that will take the strain – something to be avoided at all costs!

While it is only natural to search out those exercises that relate specifically to your own back problem, it is better to try exercises from each section, to enhance your overall improvement. So, make sure you do some exercises for each muscle area.

The exercises are arranged in approximate order of difficulty. It is vital that you do the exercises with the correct posture, so every exercise session should start with the three postural exercises on pages 82–87.

Follow these with the warm-up and then go on to between two and five exercises from each section. Finish with one or two relaxing exercises or, if you have time, the relaxation session described on page 56.

Give yourself plenty of time for your exercise and create a pleasant environment in which to do it. Put on some quiet music, if you like, but make sure it has a slow rhythm as all Pilates exercises should be performed slowly and precisely. Wear loose, comfortable clothing and leave your feet bare. Even if you are exercising on a carpet, it is a good idea to have a yoga mat or something similar, for extra support. If you have had back pain recently, it may also be a good idea at the end of your session to have a hot bath or shower (see also page 213).

WARM-UP

Begin any exercise session with the postural exercises on pages 82–87 and the simple abdominal breathing exercise on page 88. Then continue with the following three exercises.

Knee Rocks

This is a very gentle exercise for releasing the back and unlocking tension, so a particularly good one to start with if you have had a recent attack of lower back pain. Keep your head and shoulders on the floor so they stay completely relaxed.

1. Lie on your back with your knees raised and your feet flat on the floor. Breathe in and, as you breathe out, draw your navel to your spine and raise your knees towards your chest.

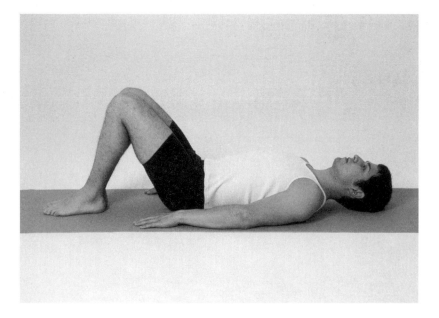

2. Place your hands just below your knees and, on the next out-breath, rock them towards you in a small, slow, gentle movement so that your lower back stretches out against the floor.

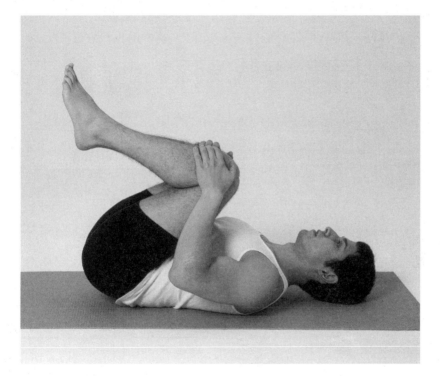

3. Do 10 slow, gentle rocks.

Head Rolls and Tilts

Many people store tension in their shoulders and necks, leading inevitably to bunched muscles, poor posture and possible side-effects such as headaches and migraines. This exercise aims to release that tension and put your spine into proper alignment.

1. Stand with a long, straight back or, if you have had recent back problems and find this uncomfortable, sit in a chair that enables you to keep your feet flat on the floor and your knees at right angles. Draw your navel gently to your spine. Check there is no tension in your shoulders, neck or face – particularly your jaw, forehead and around the eyes. Take a few long, deep breaths and let yourself relax.

2. Drop your chin down to your chest, without moving or tensing your shoulders.

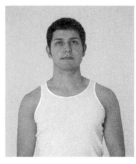 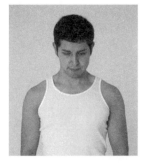

3. Roll your head around towards the left until your left ear is above your left shoulder. Slowly roll back to the centre and then continue to the right. Repeat 4–5 times on each side, checking each time that there is no tension or movement in your shoulders. Return to the central position and lift your head.

4. Now turn your head to look over your left shoulder. Keep the back of your neck long and released, and your chin slightly tucked in. Return to the centre and turn to the right. Repeat 4–5 times on each side.

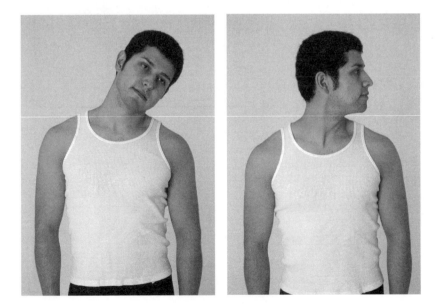

Shoulder Lifts and Circles

This exercise continues the release and mobilization of the upper body, particularly the neck, shoulders and back. Before you begin, take time to check that your body is alert but relaxed.

1. Stand or sit, as in the previous exercise, with a long straight spine. Take a few long, deep breaths and let yourself completely relax. Tilt your chin down very slightly and feel that your neck is in line with your spine.

2. Lift your shoulders up as high as you can towards your ears, letting your arms hang loosely at your sides. Let them drop down heavily, rather than placing them. Repeat 5 times. Now lift just your right shoulder 5 times, then repeat on the left.

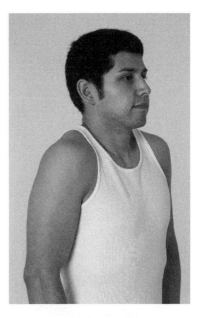

3. Draw your shoulders forwards so that you close up the front of your chest and, in a long, slow movement, circle them up towards your ears and then to the back so that you squeeze your shoulder blades together. If you feel any tension in your neck, drop your head forwards slightly. Repeat 5 times, then reverse the direction so that you start at the back and circle towards the front.

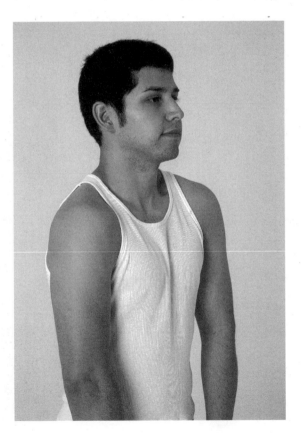

The Cossack

The best way to do this exercise is in front of a mirror so you can check your position. It is very helpful in teaching you the way your spine works and improving your posture generally, and particularly useful in mobilizing the middle back. Remember throughout to keep your spine lengthened and aligned with your navel drawn gently towards your backbone.

1. Stand squarely in front of a mirror with your arms folded a few inches in front of your chest. Rest your hands against your arms – don't grip, as this will create tension in your shoulders. Breathe in and feel your whole spine drawn gently up through the top of your head, as if you were a puppet on a string.

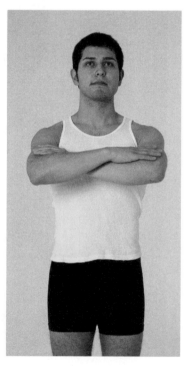

2. As you breathe out, turn – as if your spine were a pivot – feeling the turn begin at the bottom of your spine, up through your back to your shoulders and, finally, your head. Don't let your hips move – they should face straight to the front throughout.

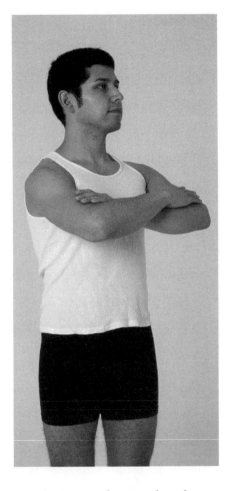

3. Breathe in and return to the starting position and, as you breathe out, turn to the other side. Alternate, 5 times on each side.

The Scoop

The scoop is a pelvic tilt that builds your awareness of and works your abdominal muscles – the most crucial muscles to strengthen to achieve a pain-free back. Make sure you begin the exercise with a neutral spine and work slowly through the base of your spine, feeling the inter-relation between your abdominal muscles and your back.

1. Lie on your back on the floor with your knees raised to the ceiling and your feet flat on the floor, hip-width apart. Check that your back is long and there is no tension in your shoulders, neck or face. Place your arms in a low V a little way from your sides.

2. Breathe in and, as you breathe out, draw your navel to your spine, squeeze the pelvic floor muscles and the low buttock muscles and feel your abdomen hollow out into a shallow scoop. This movement takes place only in the lower body – your upper body should remain still and without any tension.

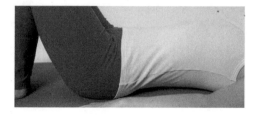

Banish Back Pain the Pilates Way

3. Repeat up to 10 times, each time trying to extend the movement. If your abdominal muscles are strong enough, you'll be able to curl your lower buttocks up very slightly from the floor. Keep your lower back on the floor at all times, though, and if you feel any strain, don't try to lift your buttocks off the floor either.

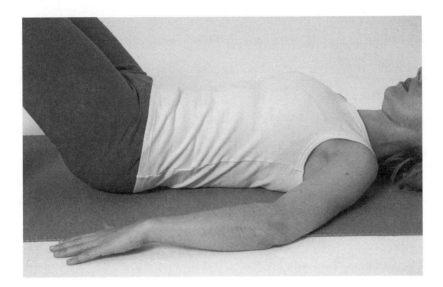

RELEASING THE UPPER AND MIDDLE BACK

The upper and middle back area includes the neck and shoulders and is one of the main areas that we tend to store tension. This tension can result in any number of distorted postures, including rigid shoulders, rounded shoulders, the head held too far forwards or back, and having one shoulder higher than the other. The latter is often the result of carrying a bag habitually on one shoulder – so it's always a good idea to swap shoulders or carry a backpack type of bag so that the weight is evenly distributed.

Muscle tension in this area frequently leads to headaches and migraines as well as backache. If the tension is not released, the muscles become increasingly rigid and postural problems and other side-effects worsen. The exercises in this section concentrate on releasing and mobilizing the upper back and correcting any poor postural habits. Even if your back problem is in your lower back, it is important to do some exercises from this section. The back is, of course, an integrated structure, and the aim of Pilates, as a holistic system, is to make the entire back function well.

Arm Stretches

These stretches bring awareness of how you should move your arms, particularly where the movement originates. When you move your arms from the middle of your back rather than by lifting the shoulders themselves, your posture improves and you are much less likely to hold tension in your back and neck.

The best way to check you are moving correctly is to do this exercise in front of a mirror. If you find the first exercise too easy, hold a can of food in each hand as a home-made weight. The added bonus with this exercise is that it simultaneously tones up your arms.

1. Stand in a relaxed posture, feet hip-width apart. If you have recently experienced back pain, you may find it easier to sit on a chair with your feet flat on the floor with a long, straight back. Draw your navel gently to your spine and pull your pelvic floor up. Check there is no tension in your shoulders, neck or face – particularly your jaw, forehead and around your eyes. Take a few long, deep breaths and let yourself relax.

2. Drop your arms down to your sides and loosely clench your fists (or hold your weights). Breathe in and, as you breathe out, slowly lift your arms straight up to the sides so they are just below shoulder level. Your arms should feel both a lift and a stretch and your shoulders should remain completely static. Repeat 5–10 times slowly.

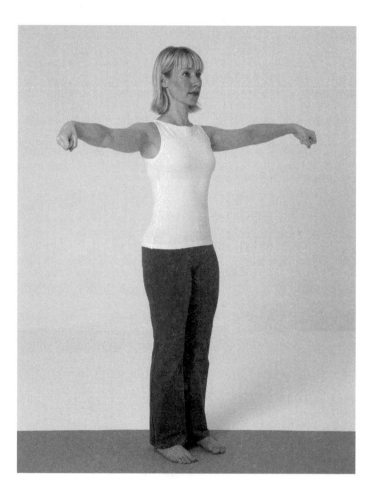

Banish Back Pain the Pilates Way

3. Drop your arms down to your sides and stretch your fingers. Breathe in and, as you breathe out, slowly take your arms behind you, keeping your palms uppermost and feeling a downward stretch in your shoulders. Go as far as you can without straining, moving your shoulders or letting the small of your back hollow out. Repeat 5–10 times slowly.

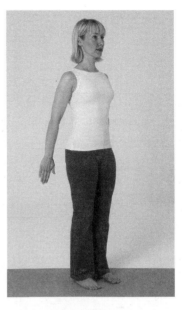

4. Bend your arms at the elbows, your fingers pointing straight ahead of you. Breathe in and open your hands out to the sides, keeping your elbows tucked in to your sides. Breathe out and return to the starting position. Repeat 5–10 times, checking there is no tension in your neck or shoulders.

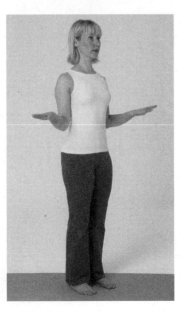

Arm Raises

This exercise helps to improve posture, as well as loosening tense necks and shoulders. You will need a long scarf or a light bamboo pole.

1. Stand with your feet hip-width apart with a long straight back and neck. Draw your navel gently towards your spine to eliminate any over-arching, and keep that feeling there throughout the exercise. Hold the scarf lightly taut with your hands about 3 feet apart.

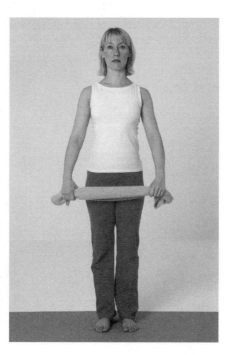

2. Breathe in and, as you breathe out, raise the scarf until it is above your head, without allowing a hollow to appear in your lower back. Don't lift your shoulders as you raise your arms. Instead, feel the movement coming from your shoulder blades. Keep your neck and shoulders soft and relaxed throughout.

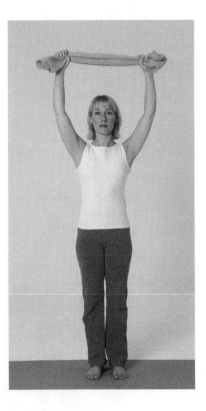

3. At the top, breathe in; then, as you breathe out, lower the scarf. Repeat 5 times.

Standing Side Stretch

This simple stretch works several different areas. It helps improve posture, uses the girdle of strength and stretches out the whole of the upper body. You need a firm support to hold on to – a heavy table or chair, for instance.

1. Stand side-on to your support with your hand resting gently on it. Start by standing close to the support for a gentle stretch, then as you become stronger and more supple, move further away for a greater stretch. Place your feet hip-width apart, check there is no tension anywhere in your body, and take a few deep breaths and try to feel yourself growing taller by lengthening your spine so you can feel space between your ribs.

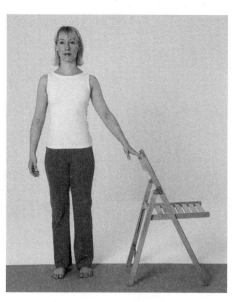

2. Breathe in and, as you breathe out, draw your navel to your spine and lift your outer arm in a wide circle up and over your head. Make sure you are facing forward the whole time and don't let your hips or shoulders turn to face the support. You should feel a stretch all the way through your side.

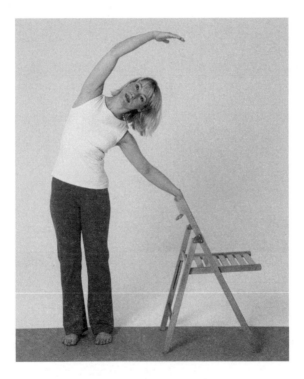

3. Breathe in to return to the starting position, checking that there is no tension in your upper body and that your shoulders are dropped. Repeat up to 10 times on both sides.

Side Stretches with Arms

This exercise works on the same principle as the last one, but is somewhat harder to do. Don't attempt it unless you can do the previous one with ease. It stretches you out sideways, but to do it correctly you must make sure that your arm moves from the centre of your back, and not from your shoulder. It is important to keep your hips and whole upper body facing directly forwards throughout.

1. Stand with your feet hip-width apart and slightly turned out, with a long, straight back and relaxed shoulders. Breathe in and, as you breathe out, draw your navel to your spine and lift up out of your waist.

2. Let your right hand start to slide down your right leg, trying to retain the feeling of lift in the ribs. Reach as far as you can, feeling the stretch up the left side of your body and taking care to keep facing square to the front.

3. Breathe in and, as you breathe out, come up and repeat 5 times on each side.

4. If you find this exercise easy, you can go on to the next stage. Stand as before, this time with your left hand on your waist. Breathe in and, as you breathe out, draw your navel to your spine and lift up out of your waist. Raise your right arm above your head.

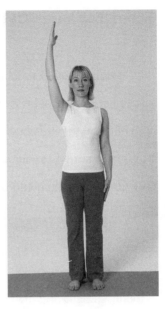

5. Bend your upper body to the left, as before, taking your right arm with you and stretching it out beyond your head. Keep your upper arm close to the side of your face and take care to keep facing square to the front.

6. Breathe in and, as you breathe out, return to the starting position. Repeat up to 5 times on each side.

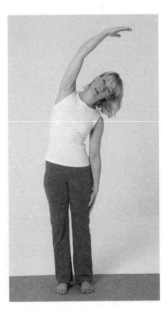

Sitting Forward Stretch

This exercise stretches and releases the back muscles, but you must be sure to keep your back straight. It is much more important to have a straight spine than to reach a lower angle. If you can only reach slightly forwards from upright, do this and gradually ease your back down over time. If you wish, you can loop a scarf around your feet to increase the stretch.

1. Sit up with a long straight spine and your legs in front of you on the floor, knees facing the ceiling and toes pointed. Relax your upper body, draw your navel to your spine and engage the buttock muscles – you should grow taller by about 2 inches!

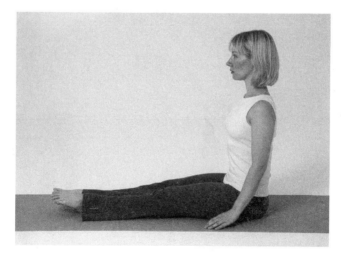

Banish Back Pain the Pilates Way

2. Breathe in and, as you breathe out, hinge at the hip sockets so that
    you reach forwards over your legs, the top of your head leading the
    way. Try not to let your shoulders tense up or your back round. This
    is a long, slow stretch and it's better to keep the length in your back
    rather than try to get as low as possible.

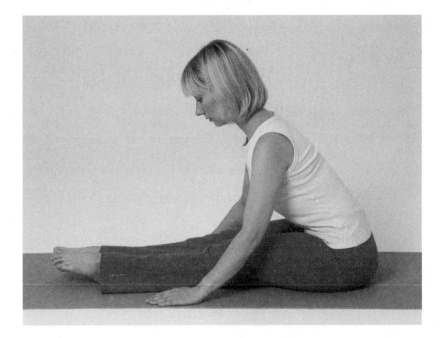

3. On the next out-breath, try to release your lower back more so that
    you reach a little further. Repeat over the next four or five out-
    breaths, each time taking the stretch a little further.

Shoulder Release

This is an excellent way of releasing tension in the shoulders, but don't strain to get your fingers clasped as that will undo any possible benefit. Instead use a scarf or belt and your shoulders will loosen over time. You will probably find one side is much looser than the other.

1. Kneel down so you are sitting on your heels with a long, straight back. Breathe in and, as you breathe out, draw your navel to your spine and release any tension in your shoulders and neck.

2. Take your scarf or belt in your right hand and stretch your right arm up to the ceiling, then bend it at the elbow so your right hand reaches down behind your neck, the scarf or belt hanging down your back.

3. Reach your left arm behind your back so that your left hand catches hold of the scarf or belt as close as it can to your right hand. Hold this position for several long, slow breaths, trying to release your shoulders more. If you can touch the fingers of your two hands together easily, you can dispense with the scarf or belt and simply clasp your fingers together. Repeat on the other side.

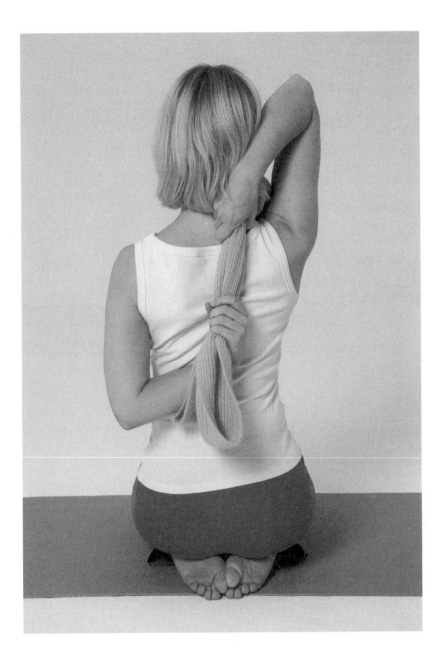

Exercises to Strengthen and Support Your Back 103

Windmill Arms

This exercise increases flexibility in the back. If you have had recent back pain, take it slowly and don't strain to reach too far. It is important to keep your spine long throughout and to keep your chest open with no tension in your neck or shoulders. This exercise also strengthens your abdominal muscles and stretches out your hamstrings.

1. Sit on the floor with a long, straight back, your neck and shoulders relaxed and your legs extended out in front of you, feet flexed, as wide as you can without feeling a strain. Remember, when you start to move the stretch will be extended. Engage your abdominal muscles so that your back is supported.

2. Breathe in and, keeping your back long and your neck and shoulders relaxed, lift your arms until they are at shoulder height, fingertips stretching away from you. Rather than lifting your shoulders to do this, try to keep them level. Instead, feel your shoulder blades drawing down into your back.

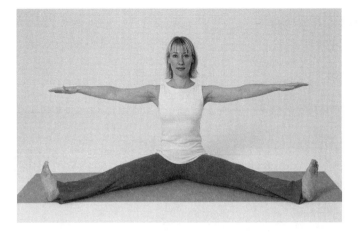

3. Breathe out and, keeping your hips and legs exactly where they are, twist your upper body to the right, controlling the movement with your abdominal muscles.

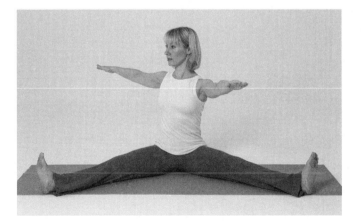

4. Reach your left hand towards your right foot, but keep the feeling of lift in the upper body – don't collapse over your legs to reach the foot.

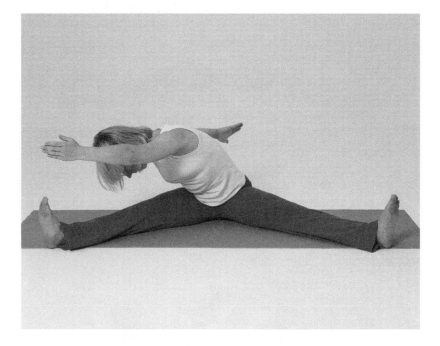

5. Breathe in to return to upright and then twist to the left, taking your right hand towards your left foot. Keep the movement smooth and lifted, and your breathing even. Repeat 5 times on each side.

Chest Stretch

This exercise is adapted from yoga and you should feel a really good stretch. If you feel any pain stop immediately, and only bend as far as you feel comfortable.

1. Stand in a good posture, shoulders relaxed, navel drawn lightly towards your spine. Take two long, slow breaths, checking there is no tension anywhere in your body. Clasp your hands loosely behind you.

2. On the next out-breath, draw your navel more firmly to your spine and, without allowing the small of your back to arch, slowly raise your hands by squeezing your shoulder blades together.

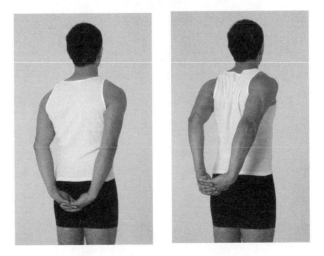

3. When you have raised your hands as far as they will comfortably go, keeping a firm hold on your abdominal muscles, bend your body forward, dropping your head towards the floor. You may find that this will release your back so that your arms stretch further.

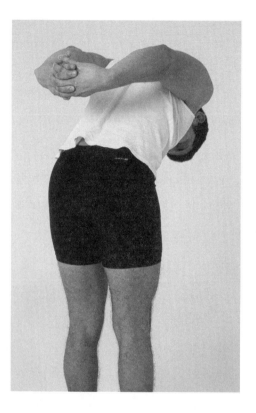

4. Hold the stretch for a few moments, then roll up slowly, vertebra by vertebra until you are back in the upright position. Do a few shoulder circles to recover.

Banish Back Pain the Pilates Way

Rib Isolations

This exercise is adapted from contemporary dance, but incorporates Pilates principles. It may seem a small movement, especially at first when you are not used to moving in this way, but it is very effective at mobilizing and stretching out the back. For maximum stretch, remember to lift up out of your hips before every movement. And, above all, *don't move your hips.* If you can, do this exercise in front of a mirror to check that your whole body remains facing forwards throughout and neither your hips nor your shoulders lift up with the movement. This is the essence of the exercise – your ribs are isolated (hence the name) and move alone.

1. Stand very tall with a long, straight back, head held in line with your spine. Check there is no tension in your neck or shoulders. Place your feet, slightly apart, directly under your hips and place your hands on your waist. Breathe in and, as you breathe out, draw your navel to your spine and gently tuck your pelvis under you. Hold this position throughout.

2. Breathe in and lift up out of your ribs, trying to feel the spaces open up between them. As you breathe out, take your ribs over to your left, trying to keep that sense of space. This movement starts from the waist. Don't move your hips at all, they should stay level and facing square to the front. Your shoulders, too, stay level; they don't tip with the angle of your ribs.

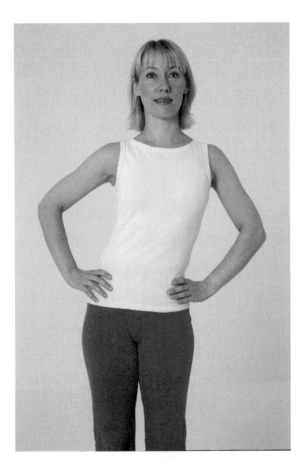

3. Breathe in and return to the centre. As you breathe out, take your ribs over to the right in the same way, so that this part of your body alone is moving. Repeat 10 times from side to side.

4. When you can do the first part of the exercise with ease, extend it by making a circle with your ribs. Move first to the left, then take your ribs to the back. You will need to do a 'scoop' to do this, exaggerating the pelvic tilt and drawing your navel to your spine more firmly. Then lengthen your spine out again as you move to the right. Finally, circle your ribs to the front, leading with your chest and remembering to keep your shoulders soft. Do 4 circles then reverse the movement.

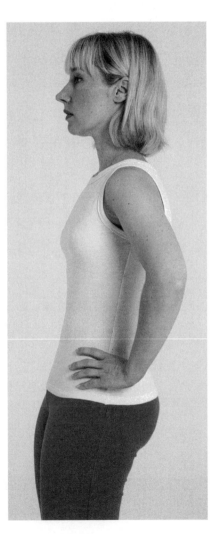

Exercises to Strengthen and Support Your Back   **111**

STRENGTHENING THE SUPPORTING MUSCLES

The underlying cause of many bad backs is not a problem with your spine itself but with the muscles that support it. These muscles include those in the back, the buttocks, legs and, most important of all, the abdominal muscles. If the abdominal muscles are not strong enough, then they cannot give the lower back the support that it needs. This makes it more likely you will arch your back and so become increasingly vulnerable to strain and injury. Strong abs are essential to good posture, and probably the single greatest protection for the back.

Pilates does not try to strengthen the abdominal muscles with sit-ups or crunches. Unfortunately, if your abdominal muscles are weak, these kinds of exercises simply put the strain on to your back – and this is the last thing you want! Instead, the focus is on awareness of these muscles, how to use them as a protection for your back as a vital part of correct posture and – having learned how to use them properly – strengthening them without compromising your back.

Pelvic Tilts

This exercise works on the Pilates girdle of strength. It builds on the
Scoop (see page 88), but you now have your feet raised up on a chair.
Always use the Scoop as a warm-up for this one and start with just
one or two repetitions, building up gradually. It is important that you
don't try to come up too far. If your lower back begins to arch or your
abdominal or thigh muscles quiver, your muscles are not yet strong
enough and you should come back down to the floor. Try it instead
with your feet flat on the floor until your abdominal muscles get
stronger. Keep the movement slow and controlled throughout.

1. Lie on your back on the floor with your feet on a stable chair.
   Check that your back is long and straight and there is no tension
   in your shoulders, neck or face. Place your arms in a low V shape,
   a little apart from your sides, with your palms facing down.

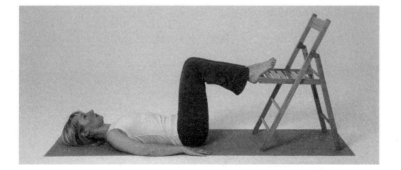

2. Breathe in and, as you breathe out, draw your navel to your spine, squeeze your pelvic floor muscles and low buttock muscles and feel your abdomen hollow out into a shallow scoop. This movement takes place only in the lower body – your upper body should remain still and free from tension.

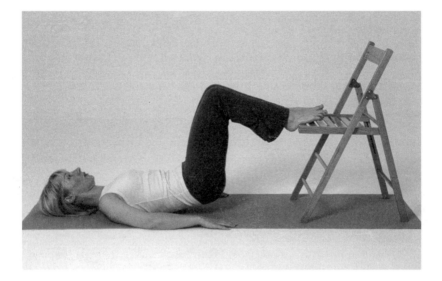

3. Keeping this scooped-out shape, curl your lower buttocks up from the floor. Repeat up to 10 times.

The Cobra

This is not the same as the yoga Cobra exercise – so you do not arch your spine to look up at the ceiling. This exercise strengthens the muscles of the back as well as the abdominal and lower buttock muscles.

1. Lie face-down on the floor with your feet slightly apart and your hands level with your forehead, palms and elbows on the floor. Breathe in and, as you breathe out, draw your navel to your spine, engaging the muscles in the lowest part of your buttocks and your pelvic floor.

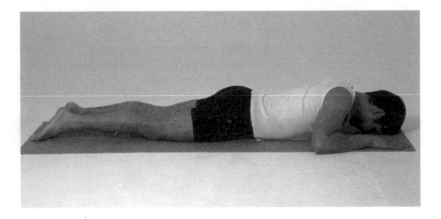

2. Draw your shoulders and the muscles of your upper back down, and at the same time lift your head off the floor, keeping your chest open. Keep your head in line with your spine – don't try to look up at the ceiling – and put as little pressure as possible on your hands and arms.

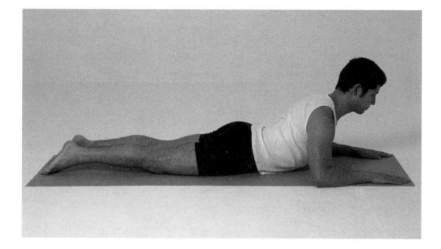

3. Breathe in to return to the starting position. Repeat up to 10 times.

Ankle Circles

You can control the amount of effort needed – according to how strong your abdominal muscles are – in this exercise. If you feel any strain in your back, raise your leg higher from the floor and the exercise becomes automatically easier. It is harder work than it looks, though, for the abdominal muscles. It is only these muscles that should be doing the work, so if you still feel a strain in your back, stop immediately.

1. Lie on your back on the floor with your shoulders and neck relaxed and your pelvis in the neutral position. Breathe in and, as you breathe out, draw your navel to your spine and lift your left leg a few inches off the floor. If this puts a strain on your back, lift it higher until you find a position that you can sustain. Point the toe.

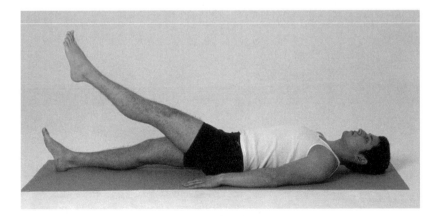

2. Make 5 slow, small and precise clockwise circles with your pointed toe, keeping your hips immobile and your knee facing the ceiling throughout – so you don't turn out your leg from the hip at any point.

3. Now make 5 anti-clockwise circles, again keeping the pelvis stable. Repeat on the other leg.

Low Leg Lifts

This exercise works in a similar way to the last one, but because the leg is low throughout, it is very hard work on the abdominal muscles, particularly in the second stage when you lift up your head. If you feel the strain in your back at any stage, stop immediately and come back to this one as your abs get stronger.

1. Lie on your back on the floor with your shoulders and neck relaxed and your pelvis in the neutral position. Your legs should be together, long and stretched out, with your toes pointed.

2. Breathe in and, as you breathe out, draw your navel to your spine and lift your left leg a few inches off the floor, without lifting your hip or displacing your pelvis. Flex your foot.

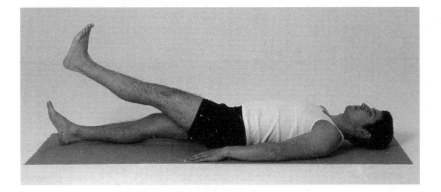

3. On the next out-breath, draw your navel firmly to your spine and lift your head and – if you can – your shoulders off the floor to look at your raised foot. Then lower both your foot and head simultaneously. If you feel any strain in your back, stop immediately.

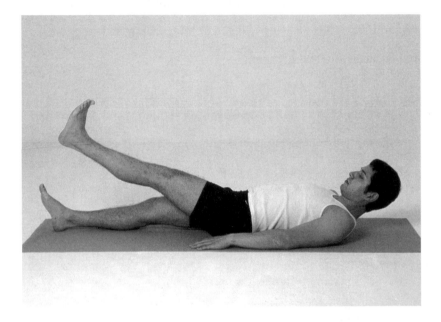

4. Repeat with your right foot and alternate up to 5 times on each side.

Can-Can

This is a lot more controlled than a real can-can – you carefully place rather than throw your legs in the air. Check that your upper body is still and does not tense up with the movement – if necessary, you can stop and check this each time you change legs. Go as slowly as you can, and take care not to distort your hips.

1. Lie on the floor with a flat back and your knees raised. Check that your hips are completely square and there is no tension in your upper body.

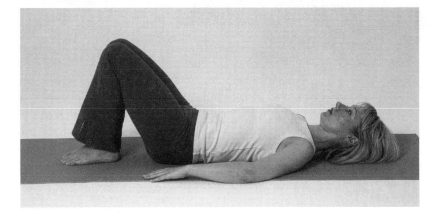

2. Breathe in and, as you breathe out, draw your navel to your spine and raise your feet so that just your toes are resting on the floor.

3. On the next out-breath, lift your left leg so that your toes point upwards but your knees are still together. This is a very slow, precise movement and it takes place in the leg – don't distort your hips to help the lift.

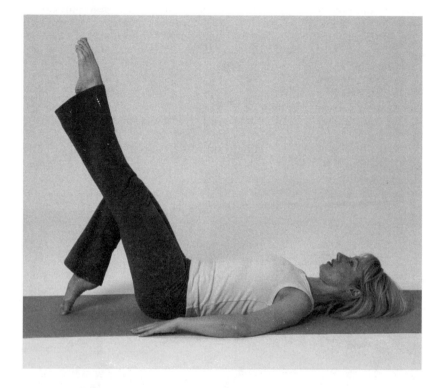

4. Replace the left leg and lift the right. Repeat slowly 5 times on each leg.

Curl-ups

This exercise is the opposite of the Scoop – it is the top of your spine rather than the bottom that moves. However, you move by using the abdominal muscles in just the same way, strengthening and placing them against your spine. This is *not* a crunch, remember. It is a very slow, controlled movement. As ever, if you feel any strain in your back or if there is any quivering or bulging out of the abdominal muscles, stop.

1. Lie on your back with your knees raised, your feet slightly apart and flat on the floor. Place a rolled-up towel or a tennis ball between your knees and keep it in place by squeezing your thighs together throughout the exercise. This will help you to retain the correct alignment and not distort your hips. Feel your spine long and relaxed. Tuck your chin in a little to release and lengthen the back of your neck. Check that your shoulders and neck are relaxed, too. Place your hands on the front of your thighs.

2. Take a long, slow breath in and, as you breathe out, draw your navel gently towards your spine and squeeze the low buttock and the pelvic floor muscles. Walk your fingers up the front of your thighs so that your head, neck and upper back start to curl up from the floor, very slowly, vertebra by vertebra. Lead with the top of your head and don't lift off any further than your shoulder blades – they should stay in contact with the floor. At the furthest point, which should be a gentle curve, check that your shoulders and neck are still relaxed and your abdominal muscles have not popped out or started to tremble.

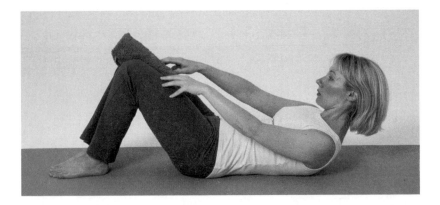

3. When you have lifted up as far as is comfortable, take another in-breath and, as you breathe out, lower your back down in exactly the same way, trying to feel each vertebra as you place it on the floor. Repeat 5–10 times, according to the strength of your abdominals.

Banish Back Pain the Pilates Way

Oblique Curl-ups

This exercise works on the same principle as the previous one, except that it uses the abdominal muscles at the sides rather than the centre of your body. You may find this exercise harder than the last one, as these muscles are used less often than the central ones, so come up only as far as you can without straining. If your abdominal muscles pop out or start to tremble, or if you feel back pain at any time, stop immediately.

1. Lie on your back as in the previous exercise, with a rolled-up towel or a tennis ball between your knees. As before, keep it in place by squeezing your inner thighs together throughout the exercise to keep correct alignment. Place your hands just behind your ears – but don't use your arms to pull your head or shoulders up from the floor. Your shoulders and neck should stay relaxed throughout – check each time you start to curl up.

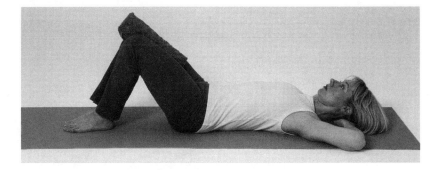

2. Breathe in and, as you breathe out, draw your navel gently to your spine and start to curl your head and neck up, turning your body so that your right shoulder points towards your left knee. Don't lead with your elbow – keep your elbows wide, your chest open and your shoulders soft. Move slowly and go only so far as you can without your abdominal muscles bulging or trembling.

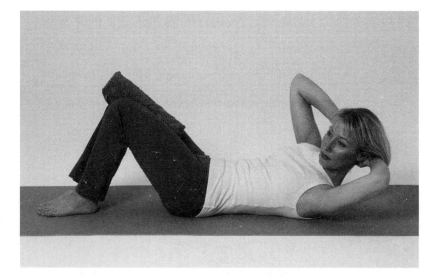

3. Breathe in and, on the out-breath, curl back down to the floor. Relax for a moment, check there is no tension (particularly in your neck or shoulders), then repeat to the other side, curling your left shoulder towards your right knee. Repeat, alternating from side to side, up to 5 times.

Banish Back Pain the Pilates Way

Reverse Curl-ups

The reverse curl-up is harder for most people than the previous two exercises, and the abdominal muscles have to work very hard. It is a small movement, so don't strain to go too far and, if you feel the strain at any time, stop.

1. Lie on your back with your feet flat on the floor, your head, neck and shoulders relaxed. Take a long breath in and, as you breathe out, draw your navel to your spine and bring your legs up so that your knees form a right angle. Cross your feet at your ankles.

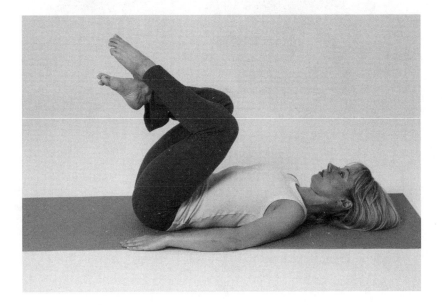

2. Breathe in and, as you breathe out, engage the abdominal muscles, squeeze your buttock muscles and lift your bottom off the floor, at the same time as your head and shoulders come up to meet your knees.

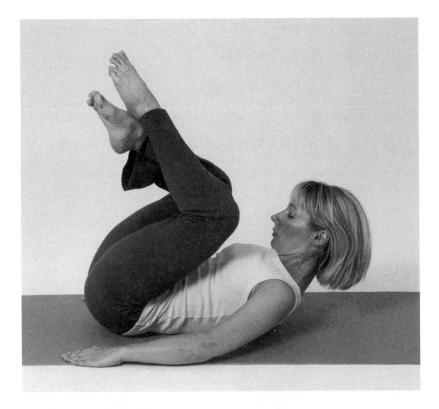

3. Relax your head down to the floor and your knees back to the right-angle position. Repeat up to 10 times.

Roll-ups

This exercise is excellent for building up abdominal strength, but only if your abdominal muscles are already quite toned up. It should always be done in a smooth and controlled way – in fact, the more slowly you do it, the harder it is. If you find the effort goes into your back or neck, your abs aren't yet strong enough. Concentrate on other exercises and leave this one until you're ready.

1. Lie on your back with your feet flat on the floor, your knees bent, your pelvis in 'neutral' and your upper body relaxed. Breathe in and lift your arms and take them above your head and down on to the floor behind you so your fingertips and toes are now pointing away from each other in a long stretch.

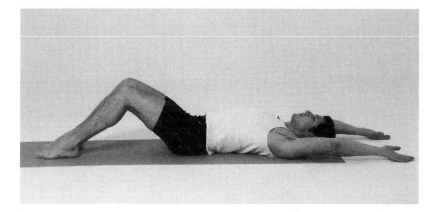

2. On the next in-breath, raise your arms to point straight up to the ceiling.

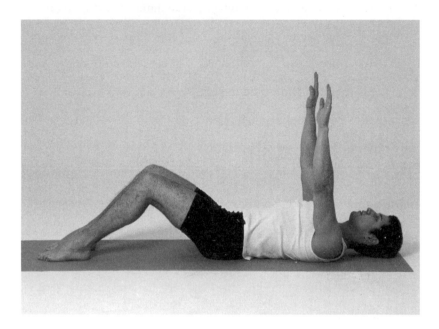

3. As you breathe out, draw your navel to your spine and engage your low buttock muscles. Starting with your head, your chin dropped to the chest, start to roll up slowly into a sitting position. The movement should be slow and controlled, with no tension in your shoulders, back or neck. (If there is, or if your abdominal muscles start to bulge out or quiver, they aren't strong enough – release back down to the floor.)

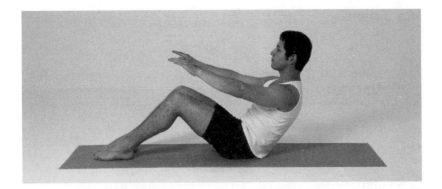

4. Keep your arms extended out in front of you as you roll forward, keeping your abdominal muscles working hard, your navel drawn towards your spine, so there is a rounded curve in your lower back. This will stop you collapsing over your legs as you reach forward.

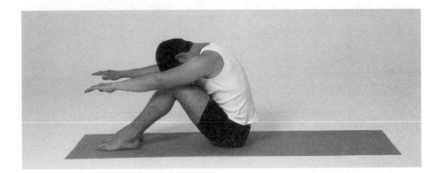

5. When you have reached your full extent, breathe in and, as you breathe out, roll back up to a sitting position. Breathing out, continue down to the floor again in one long, slow, controlled movement. Repeat up to 4 times.

Exercises to Strengthen and Support Your Back   **131**

Hip Balance

This exercise is all about abdominal strength. The movement itself is actually very small, but also very controlled. The back is rounded so you should not feel any strain but, if you do, stop immediately.

1. Sit with your feet flat on the floor, knees close to your chest. Stretch out your fingers and place your hands so that your thumbs are against your chest and your little fingers are against your thighs. Your aim is to keep your fingers stretched out and the same distance between your chest and thighs throughout the exercise.

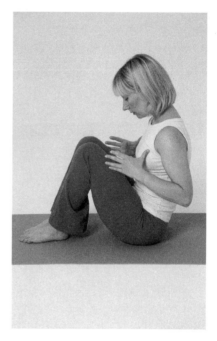

2. Breathe in and, as you breathe out, draw your navel to your spine and curve your back, taking your feet just off the floor.

3. Keeping the same hand span distance between thighs and chest, rock back on your buttocks as far as you can without losing your balance. You will need to hold on firmly with your abdominal muscles.

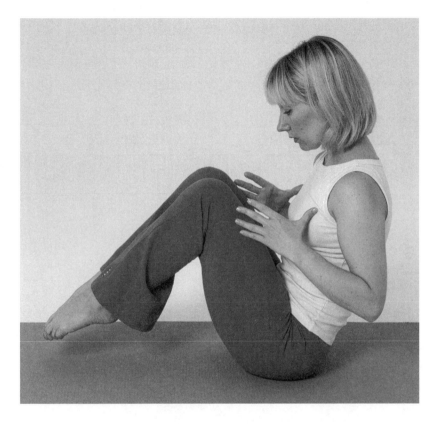

4. Move between these two positions slowly and smoothly, your abdominal muscles controlling the movement. Repeat up to 10 times.

Leg Stretches

This is one of the most famous of Pilates' exercises, though in a somewhat gentler version to try to avoid straining the back. It is an excellent exercise for strengthening the abdominal muscles. You can control the amount of effort by raising or lowering your legs. The higher they are, the easier the exercise becomes, so in this version they point straight up to the ceiling. However, as your muscles become stronger you can try lowering your legs slightly to increase the effort. The effort should, though, be entirely in your abdominal muscles, leaving your upper body, particularly your neck and shoulders, soft and relaxed. If you feel any strain in your back, stop immediately.

1. Lie on your back with your feet flat on the floor and your knees raised. Now draw your knees to your chest, keeping them apart to make a V-shape towards your toes. Check that your back is flat on the floor and your neck and shoulders are relaxed.

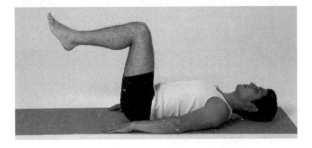

2. Breathe in and bring one knee up towards your chest. Then, as you breathe out, draw your navel to your spine, making sure your whole spine is on the floor, and stretch the second leg vertically up into the air with a pointed toe. Check that your spine is still elongated along the floor and there is no tension in your neck or shoulders.

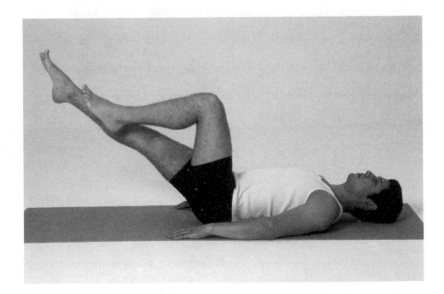

3. Take another long full breath and, as you breathe out, change legs so the second leg is drawn in towards the chest and the first is stretched out. Always keep your whole back on the floor. If you start to hollow out the small of your back, your leg is too low – make sure it is 90 degrees to the floor. If you feel any discomfort, stop immediately. Alternate 5–10 times on each side.

Exercises to Strengthen and Support Your Back   **135**

Double Leg Stretch

The double leg stretch is one of the most famous – and tough – Pilates' sequential movements. Here it is adapted to avoid putting a strain on your back. It's not too easy, though, as your abdominal muscles have to be strong enough to carry the weight of both your legs. Make sure you stretch your legs upwards at 90 degrees to the floor – the lower your legs, the harder the exercise is to do and, as with the previous exercise, you can adapt it to make it harder as you become stronger. Keep checking that your abdominals aren't bulging out or trembling with the effort. If they do either, stop immediately.

1. Lie on your back with your knees bent, feet flat on the floor and your back long and straight. Place your hands, with your fingers lightly clasped, behind your head. Don't use your hands to pull your head up, though, and keep checking throughout that your shoulders and neck are free from tension.

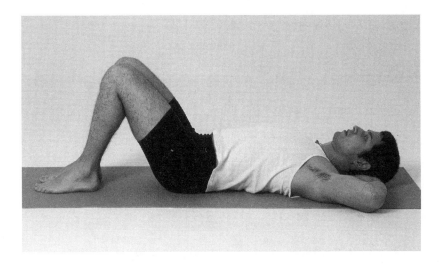

2. Breathe in and, as you breathe out, draw your navel to your spine and bend your knees to a right angle, feet softly pointed.

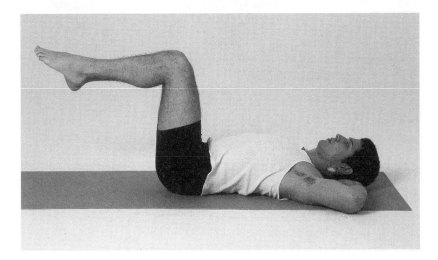

3. On the next out-breath, curl your head and neck up from the floor – keep checking that your abdominal muscles are working – and simultaneously straighten your legs up towards the ceiling. If it is uncomfortable to straighten your legs completely, you can leave your knees slightly bent.

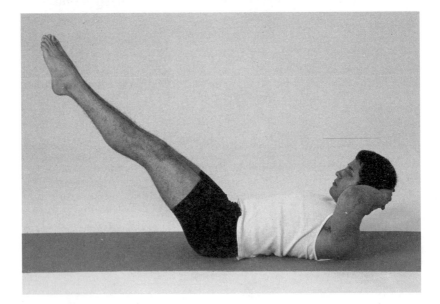

4. Breathe in and, as you breathe out, bend your knees back to right angles and lower your head to the floor. Check for any tension. Repeat up to 10 times.

The Hundred

Another classic – and notoriously difficult – Pilates exercise. This is a
simplified version but, even so, you should build up to it gradually.
Don't expect to get to 100 taps the first time you do it, and watch out
for warning signs – bulging abdominals or back strain – that you are
doing too much. If either occurs, stop immediately.

1. Lie on your back with your knees raised, feet flat on the floor and
   your arms relaxed by your sides. Check there is no tension in your
   neck or shoulders, placing a small pillow under your head if that
   makes you more comfortable. Breathe in and, as you breathe out,
   draw your navel to your spine and raise your legs so that your
   knees are bent and your calves are parallel to the floor. Gently
   point your toes.

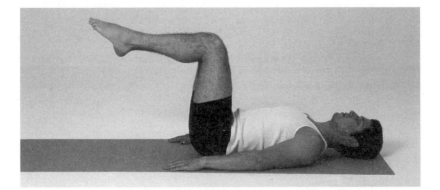

2. Keeping your legs in the same position throughout, breathe in and, as you breathe out, raise your head to look at your knees. With your arms parallel, make five taps on the floor on the next inhalation, then five more taps on the exhalation.

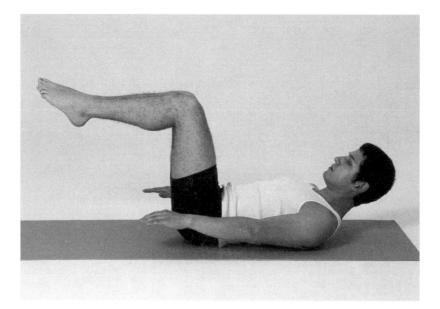

3. Breathe slowly and evenly and continue the taps in time with the breath, aiming for 100 taps in all. If at any time you feel strain in your back, shoulders or neck, stop.

4. Draw your knees to your chest and hug them for a few moments, rocking your back gently from side to side to iron out any tension.

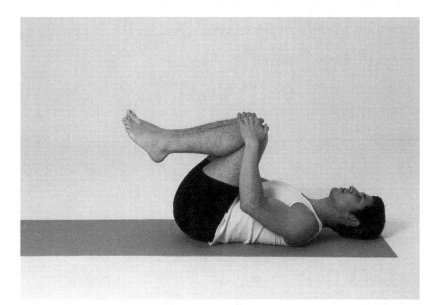

Forward Leg Lifts

This is another strengthening exercise for the abdominal muscles. Both versions are difficult – the second more so than the first! Whichever one you do, it is important to keep lifting out of your waist – don't let yourself slump down towards the floor. As always, if you feel any strain in the back, stop immediately.

1. Lie on your right side in a long straight line, your head resting on your right arm. If you wish, you can place a small cushion or a rolled-up towel underneath your waist to remind you to keep it lifted. Check that your legs are exactly together, without one foot extending further than the other. Check, too, that there is no tension in your neck or shoulders, and keep checking throughout the exercise.

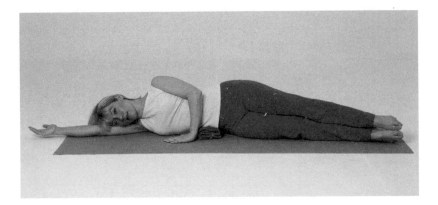

2. Breathe in and, as you breathe out, draw your navel to your spine, tilt your pelvis slightly forwards and lift your legs about an inch off the floor. Check that there is still no tension in your upper body.

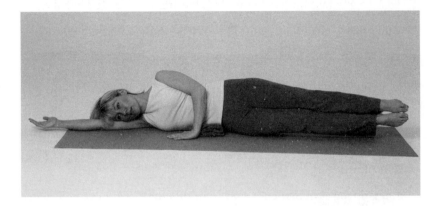

3. Keeping your lower leg off the floor, raise the top leg a few inches further.

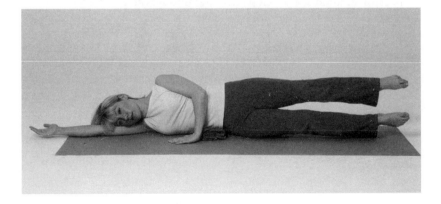

4. Bring the raised leg out to the front in a slow movement without distorting your pelvis. Raise and lower 10 times. Repeat on the other side. If you find this easy after a while, you can make it more challenging by sitting on your hip, with your hands used to balance you – not to take the weight off your legs, though. Sit on your right hip, legs straight out to the side. Place your right hand on the floor as a balance and lift up out of your ribs, lengthening your body.

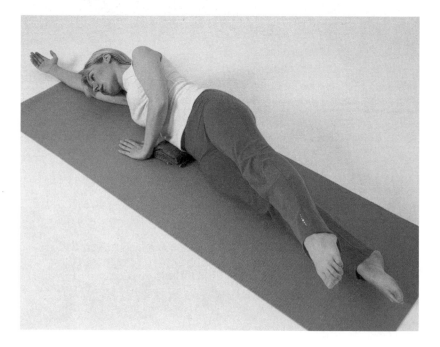

5. Breathe in and, as you breathe out, draw your navel to your spine, tilt your pelvis slightly forwards and lift your legs about an inch off the floor. Check that there is still no tension in your upper body.

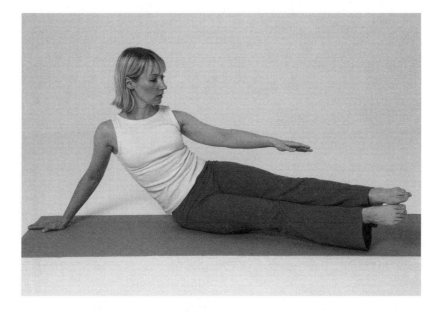

6. Keeping your lower leg off the floor, raise the top leg a few inches further and take it out in front of you in a slow movement without distorting your pelvis. Raise and lower 10 times. Repeat on the other side.

Buttock Squeeze

This exercise tones – and helps you locate – a major part of the Pilates girdle of strength: the lower abdominal and buttock muscles. Strengthening these muscles is vital to protect the back. Take care not to arch in the lower back or let any tension creep into the back, neck or shoulders. In fact, the top part of the body should be completely relaxed throughout.

1. Lie face-down on the floor with a pillow underneath your abdomen and a smaller one between your thighs. Rest your forehead on your hands, turning your head to one side if that is more comfortable. Your shoulders and neck should be relaxed.

2. Breathe in and, as you breathe out, draw your navel off the cushion, pressing it back towards your spine and, at the same time, squeeze the cushions between your thighs using the muscles at the base of your buttocks and inner thighs. Hold for a count of 5–10 and release. Check that there is no tension in your upper body and repeat up to 5 times.

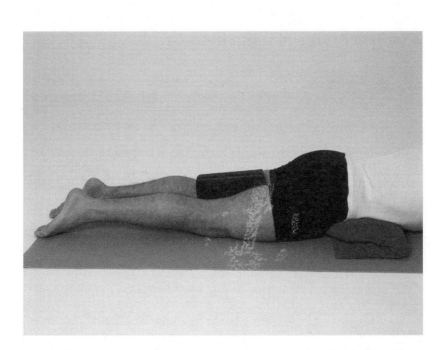

Alternate Arms and Legs Stretches

This exercise works not only on the Pilates' central girdle of strength, it tones and stretches the arms and legs, as well. The pillow is used to remind you to keep lifting your abdominal muscles away from the floor – when you are stronger, you'll see that a gap will open up between you and the cushion.

1. Lie face-down with a cushion beneath your abdominal muscles. With your feet hip-width apart, knees facing the floor, stretch your arms above your head, palms facing the floor. Check that your shoulders and neck are relaxed. Breathe in and, as you breathe out, draw your navel to your spine and hold this position throughout the exercise.

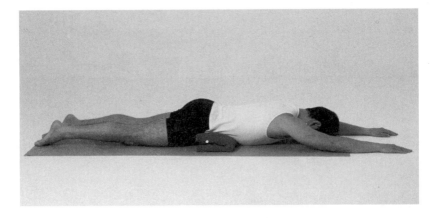

2. Breathe in and, as you breathe out, stretch your left leg and right arm as far as you can, keeping them low to the floor. When you have stretched as much as possible, breathe in and lower your arm and leg to the floor.

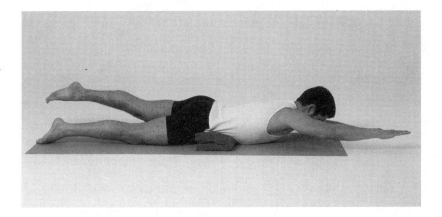

3. Breathe in and, as you breathe out, stretch the right leg and left arm as far as you can. Check that there is no tension in your neck, shoulders or jaw and that your navel is still strong and drawn to your spine. Repeat up to 5 times.

The Bridge

This exercise is a Pilates adaptation of a yoga position. It strengthens the back and buttock muscles, but you must take care not to let your back arch or this will put a strain on it. Concentrate on keeping your navel drawn towards your spine to prevent this. Try to keep your neck and shoulders relaxed throughout. If you feel any strain in your back, stop immediately.

1. Lie on your back, with your feet flat on the floor, hip-width apart. There should be no arching in the lower spine. Place your arms in a low V, a little away from your body, palms flat on the floor. Check there is no tension in your neck or shoulders.

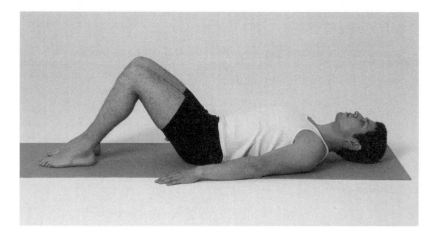

Banish Back Pain the Pilates Way

2. Breathe in and, as you breathe out, draw your navel to your spine, squeeze your buttock muscles and start to lift your buttocks and lower back from the floor. The aim is to make a long diagonal with only your shoulders and feet on the floor, but if this places too much of a strain on your back, come off the floor only as far as you can without discomfort.

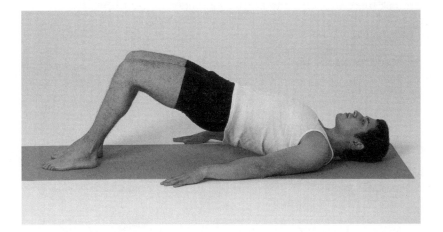

3. Hold the position for a few seconds (longer if you can), breathe in and, as you breathe out, roll your spine back to the floor, starting at the top and trying to feel each vertebra, one by one, touch the floor.

Backward Leg Lifts

Although it is natural to bend your body forwards in this exercise, you must keep your back straight throughout for maximum benefit. The key is to keep your abdominal muscles engaged, your navel drawn back to your spine throughout. This exercise will strengthen the supporting buttock muscles and, if you keep a good posture, your back, too.

1. Stand in a good posture facing the back of a heavy chair or another piece of furniture that will support your weight. Hold the chair back with both hands and check your posture. You should have a long, straight spine and there should be no tension in your neck or shoulders.

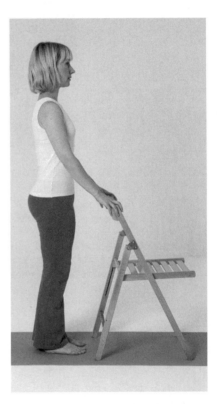

Banish Back Pain the Pilates Way

2. Breathe in and, as you breathe out, draw your navel to your spine and, keeping your back upright, slowly take your right leg out behind you, squeezing your buttock as you do so.

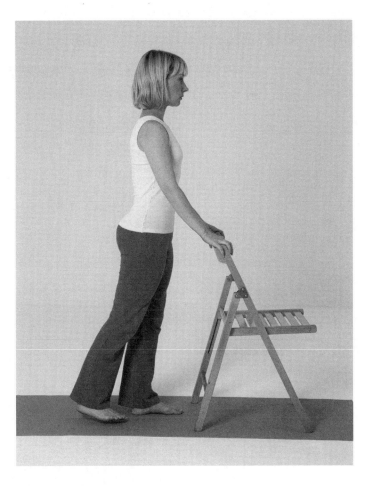

3. Do 10 lifts on each side.

MOBILIZING AND RELAXING THE BACK

Many back problems are caused or exacerbated by stiffness, tension and a general lack of mobility. Few of us use the range of movements that our backs are capable of, and so muscles become weaker and joints stiffen up. Because Pilates works on the smaller muscle groups and joints as well as the larger ones, it is one of the most effective ways of bringing movement back to your body. When the back is used fully, it is much less likely to store tension and become rigid.

There is, of course, now a recognized link between physical and mental or emotional tension. This is explored more fully in Part Four, where there are a number of techniques suggested to help you relax. In this section, the focus is on relaxing and freeing up the back from physical tension; most people find that this has a direct effect on mental and emotional stress, too. This is one of the reasons that Pilates is generally regarded as a particularly relaxing form of exercise.

Legs Against the Wall

This is an excellent position in which to relax after the more strenuous exercises. It is also a good stretch that simultaneously works the abdominal muscles, but you must keep the whole length of your back on the floor throughout. If your lower back arches or you feel any strain, stop immediately.

1. Using a cushion beneath your head, position yourself so that your bottom touches the wall. It is probably easiest to approach the wall by rolling sideways into position and bending your knees down towards your body. Check that your back is relaxed and long.

2. Walk your legs up the wall as far as is comfortable. If they stretch effortlessly, straighten your legs and flex your feet; otherwise, keep your toes pointed and your knees bent. Do not arch your lower back. If you just want to relax, hold this position for up to 5 minutes.

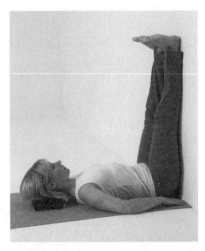

3. If you want to make this more of an exercise than a relaxation, you can add to it by creating a stretch for your inner thighs. Breathe in and, as you breathe out, draw your navel to your spine and gradually let your legs stretch outwards to the sides until you feel a stretch – but not a strain. If your lower back comes off the floor, bring your legs closer together until it is flat again. Open and close slowly up to 5 times and, if you find this comfortable, relax in this position for 5 minutes.

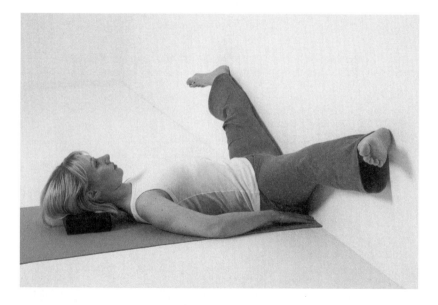

4. Bend your knees and roll sideways onto the floor to come out of either position.

Leg Slides

This exercise helps you to develop awareness of good alignment and posture if you concentrate on keeping your pelvis still and letting your leg do all the movement. It also mobilizes and stretches the joints of the leg.

1. Lie on the floor with your knees raised and feet together on the floor. Check your back and neck are aligned and elongated, with no arching in the small of your back and no tension in your shoulders.

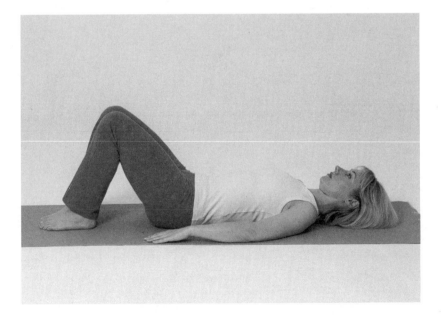

2. Breathe in and, as you breathe out, draw your navel to your spine and straighten one bent knee along the floor, without distorting your pelvis or back. Make it a long, slow stretch throughout your leg and foot, pointing your toes. Breathe in and return to the starting position. Check that you have not changed the position of your hips.

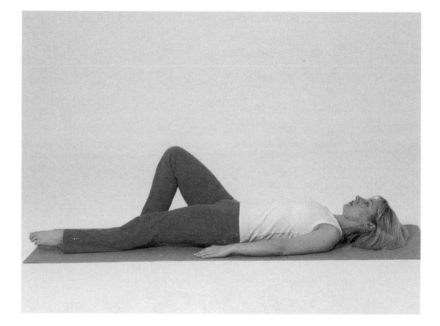

3. Repeat with the other leg on the next out-breath. Alternate 5 times on each side.

The Cat

This is a wonderful exercise for releasing tension, and is used in numerous exercise disciplines. It stretches and releases the back. The best way of doing it is as slowly and smoothly as possible, allowing one position to blend into the next. If you feel any strain, however, or have experienced any recent back pain, do only the first two positions.

1. If possible, position yourself next to a mirror so you can check that your back is completely flat. Position yourself on your hands and knees, knees hip-width apart. Check that your shoulders, hips and knees are in a straight line, like the top of a table. Try to make your back perfectly flat with no tension in your neck and your head relaxed and in line with your spine, not dropped down between your shoulders.

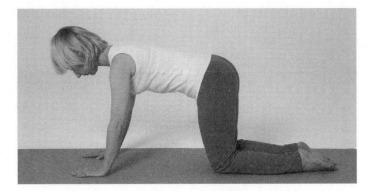

2. Breathe in and, as you breathe out, gently draw your navel back towards your spine so that your back arches upwards and your head drops down between your arms. Breathe in and return to position one.

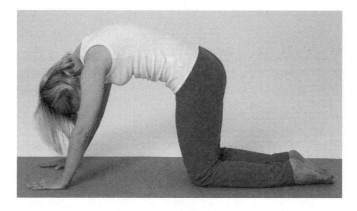

3. Breathe out and arch your back the other way, so that it hollows out, your head and your bottom the highest points of your body. Breathe in and return to position one. Repeat 5–10 times.

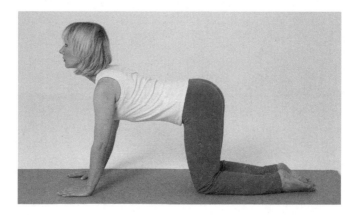

Cat with a Leg Stretch

This is a variation on the Cat exercise and it does work the abdominal muscles quite hard. Don't try it until your abs are strong. It is important not to confuse this with the exercise that you often do in aerobics classes, where you fling the leg up behind you. Instead, you should do this slowly, keeping your hips level and your back flat throughout. If you find it a strain, or if you have recently had back pain, do the original Cat instead.

1. Kneeling on all fours, elongate your spine and keep your neck in line with it. You are aiming at a completely flat, table-top back! Make sure there is no tension in your shoulders or neck. Breathe in and, as you breathe out, draw your navel to your spine and raise your left knee up towards your chest, dropping your head.

2. Breathe in and straighten your leg out behind you, raising your head – in line with your spine, not looking up towards the ceiling. Repeat up to 10 times, alternating legs each time.

Dog Pose

This is a lovely stretch for the back, releasing any tension and lengthening it out. Your aim is to keep your back as long and straight as possible, eventually by pushing back on your heels and away from your hands. However, you are unlikely to be able to do this at first, so just concentrate on lengthening out, keeping any tension out of your neck.

1. Kneeling on all fours, elongate your spine and keep your neck in line with it. Then, tuck your toes under, breathe out and draw your navel to your spine. Now, press up from the floor so that the soles of your feet are as close as you can to flat on the floor and make a triangle shape, with your bottom as the apex. Straighten your legs as far as possible, your back long, your neck and head in line with your spine. If you can, try to extend the stretch by pressing your heels to the floor and stretching away from your hands as you take long, deep breaths, checking that there is no tension in your shoulders or neck. Hold for up to 1 minute.

Banish Back Pain the Pilates Way

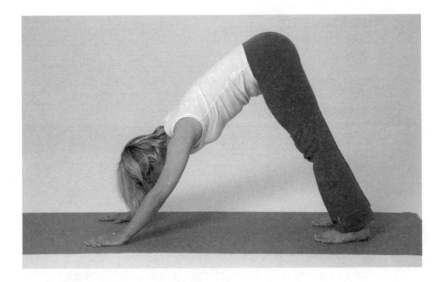

2. Drop your knees back down to the floor and then sit back on your heels, your arms stretched out in front of you – this is known as the Child's Pose. Rest your head on the floor, turning it to one side if this is more comfortable for you. Relax into this position and breathe deeply.

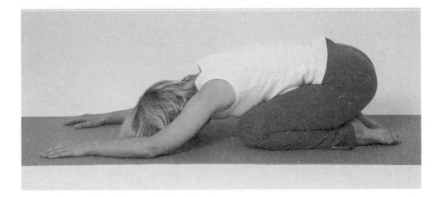

Exercises to Strengthen and Support Your Back   163

Dog Pose Sequence

This sequence of movements incorporates both the Child and the Dog poses from yoga and has a lovely, flowing momentum. Really stretch and relax into each position for maximum mobilization and release.

1. Begin in the Dog pose so that you make a triangle, your bottom as the apex. Straighten your legs as much as possible, keeping your back long and your head and neck in line with 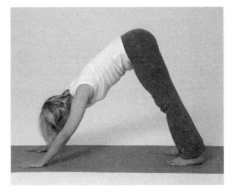 your spine. Breathe in and, as you breathe out, draw your navel to your spine and lengthen the stretch as much as you can.

2. Breathe in and, as you breathe out, drop your knees to the floor and sit back on your heels in the Child pose, arms stretched 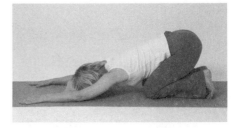 out in front of you but with no tension in your neck or shoulders.

3. Breathe in and, as you breathe out, come off your heels, stretching your body low along the floor. When your chest becomes level with your hands, turn your toes under so you are in a low press-up. If this is uncomfortable, keep your knees slightly bent and in contact with the floor.

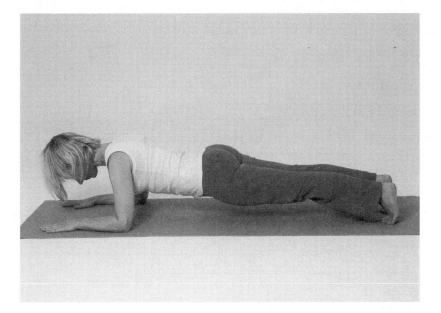

4. On the next out-breath, drop your head down towards the floor and lift your buttocks to form the Dog pose triangle again. Repeat up to 5 times.

Forward Bend

This is a long, strong stretch for the back, which opens up the vertebrae. For this exercise you need a heavy chair or another stable piece of furniture that can support your weight – make sure it won't move as you reach forward. It is very important in this exercise to keep your back long and free from tension, so make sure you reach from your back rather than your shoulders.

1. Stand with good posture, feet hip-width apart, with a long, straight back and relaxed shoulders. Position yourself at the distance from your chair that will give you a good stretch when you bend.

2. Breathe in and, as you breathe out, draw your navel to your spine and raise your arms. Engage your abdominal and buttock muscles and, keeping your back absolutely straight, bend forwards from your hips until your fingers reach the chair back. Your hips should act as a hinge – your back does not round at all as you stretch forwards. You should feel a good stretch in this position – if not, move slightly further back from the chair. Make sure that there is no tension in your shoulders, and try to pull your shoulder blades gently down your back.

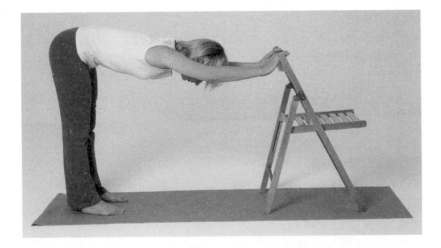

3. Hold the stretch for up to a minute, then take your fingers off the chair and let your back roll down until you are hanging upside down. Hold this position for up to a minute, then slowly roll back up, feeling each vertebra position itself into a long, straight back, your navel still drawn to your spine.

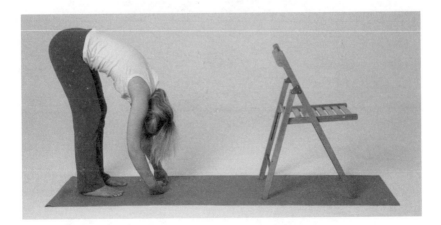

Floor Twists

This exercise gives a long, oblique stretch to the back, and is both lengthening and loosening. It is important to keep both shoulders as much as possible on the floor for the best stretch. If you have had any recent back pain, leave out the last stage where you straighten the leg, and if you feel any strain at any time, stop immediately.

1. Lie on your back on the floor with your arms out at shoulder level, neck and shoulders relaxed. Breathe in and, as you breathe out, draw your navel to your spine and raise your legs so they form a right angle at the knee.

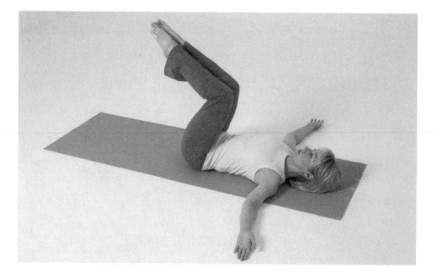

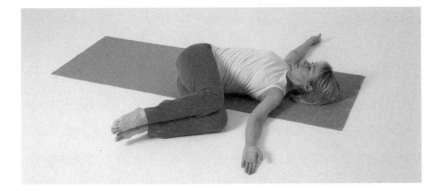

2. Keeping your abdominal muscles engaged, on the next out-breath take your knees over to the left, so the left leg is in contact with the floor, but the shoulders don't lift up.

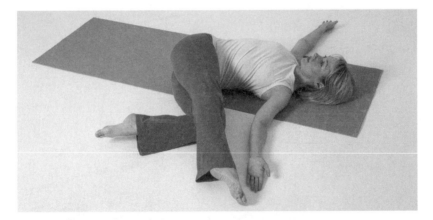

3. Keeping your knees level, stretch out your right leg and, if you can, take hold of your right toes with your left hand and try to draw the leg gently higher. Hold the stretch for up to a minute, if you can, and then repeat on the other side.

Hip Rolls

This exercise is designed to release tension from the back and neck. Your abdominal muscles are 'carrying' the weight of your legs, so don't take them so far that it puts a strain on your back or the abdominals themselves. As with any exercise that involves a twist, only go as far as you can without straining. If you feel any pain, stop immediately.

1. Lie on your back with your feet hip-width apart, your knees raised. Check that your neck and spine are relaxed and long.

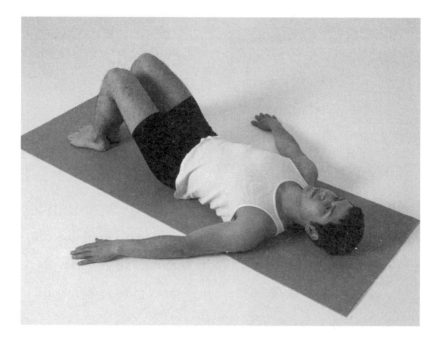

Banish Back Pain the Pilates Way

2. Breathe in and, as you breathe out, draw your navel towards your spine. Do not distort your back. Roll your knees gently to one side. Take them only as far as they will go without your buttocks coming off the floor.

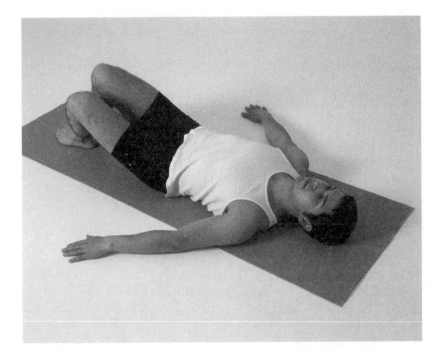

3. Breathe in to return to the centre and, as you breathe out, roll your knees to the other side. Repeat up to 10 times on each side.

Hip Isolations

This is a very similar exercise to the rib isolations on page 109, but now the movement takes place in the hips. As with the rib isolations, it is the hips alone that move, all of the rest of your body remaining still.

1. Stand very tall with a long, straight back, head held in line with your spine. Check there is no tension in your neck or shoulders. Place your feet, slightly apart, directly under your hips and place your hands on the front of your hip bones. Breathe in and, as you breathe out, draw your navel to your spine and gently tuck your pelvis under you. Hold this position throughout.

2. Breathe in and lift up out of the ribs, trying to feel the spaces open up between them. As you breathe out, squeeze your right hip up towards your waist, so that the left side of your body lengthens out. You will need to bend your knees gently, but don't move your upper body at all – your shoulders should stay level and facing square to the front.

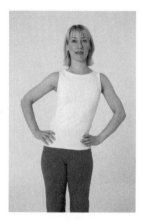

3. Breathe in and return to the centre. As you breathe out, squeeze your left hip in the same way so that this part of your body alone is moving. Repeat 10 times from side to side.

4. When you can do the first part of this exercise with ease, extend it by making a circle with your hips. Move first to the right, then take your hips to the back. This is one of the few times that you actually arch in your lower back. Then lengthen your spine out again as you move to the left. Finally, circle your hips to the front, leading with your pelvis, scooping out your abdominal muscles and remembering to keep your shoulders soft. Do 4 circles, then reverse the movement.

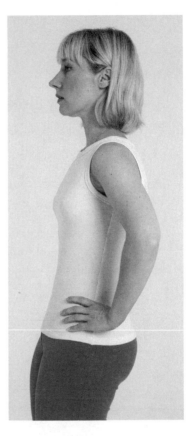

Spinal Twist

This is both a relaxing exercise for the back and a stretch for the hamstring and calf muscles. Don't overdo it, though – go just as far as the stretch, without it becoming a strain. You will need a long scarf or belt.

1. Sit up straight with a long back and relaxed shoulders. Place your right leg out straight in front of you and bend your left leg, tucking your foot into your groin. Loop the scarf around your outstretched right foot and check there is no arching in your lower back or rounding of your shoulders. Hold the scarf in your left hand.

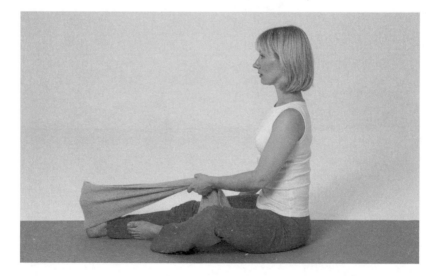

2. Without tensing your back or shoulders, stretch your right leg, foot flexed. Breathe deeply and hold the stretch for about a minute.

3. Place your right hand on the floor just behind you and, still holding the scarf in your left hand, start to turn towards your right. Your spine should stay completely vertical and you should feel as if it is a pole around which you are pivoting. Keep your sitting bones firmly on the floor and your shoulders level, and check there is no tension in your neck, shoulders or chest. Hold the stretch for up to 1 minute, breathing deeply.

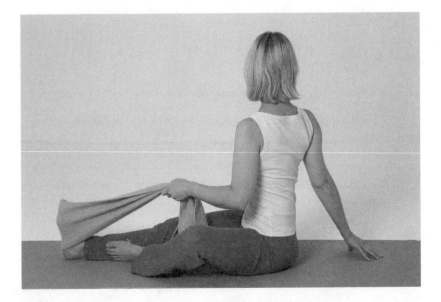

4. Turn slowly back to the centre and repeat on the left leg.

Exercises to Strengthen and Support Your Back　　　**175**

Child's Pose

This is actually a yoga pose rather than a Pilates exercise, but it is
perfect for releasing and stretching the back. Your ultimate aim is to
make your bottom sit on your heels so that the whole of your spine is
stretched out over your legs, but you won't be able to get there at first.
Strange as it may sound, if you have someone to help you it is very
relaxing if they push your buttocks down to help you to achieve this
position. Don't strain, though – this is principally a relaxation pose.

1. Kneel down on the floor and sit back as much as possible on your
    heels. Bend forwards, place your forehead on the floor, or on a
    small cushion, and stretch your arms out as flat on the floor as you
    can. Check there is no tension anywhere in your body (your neck,
    shoulders and back are all potential danger spots) and feel a stretch
    along the whole length of your spine.

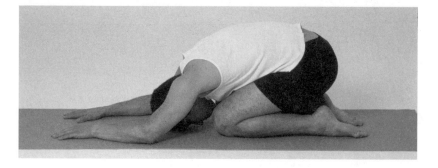

2. Take one arm back and lay it down at your side, palm uppermost. If it is more comfortable, turn your head so that your cheek rather than your forehead is against the floor.

3. Now take your other arm and lay it down next to you in the same way. Relax into the pose for 2 minutes, or longer if you have the time.

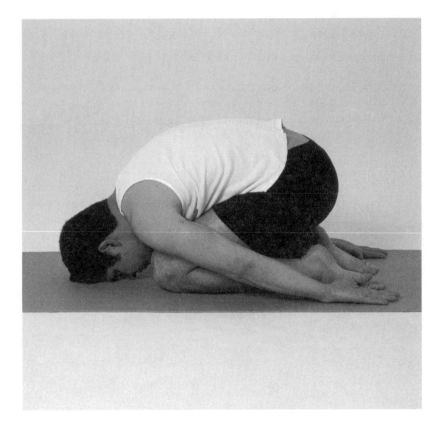

Pillow Squeeze

This well-known Pilates exercise combines several benefits; it is usually one of the last used in a Pilates session. It works the inner thighs and pelvic floor muscles, as well as helping with postural awareness and relaxing your lower back. You will need a cushion or pillow – the firmer it is, the harder you will have to work.

1. Lie on your back, knees raised, feet flat on the floor. Place your arms by your sides, palms down. Check that your neck and shoulders are relaxed. If you are uncomfortable at all or if your neck feels arched, place a small cushion beneath your head. Breathe in, pulling up your pelvic floor muscles.

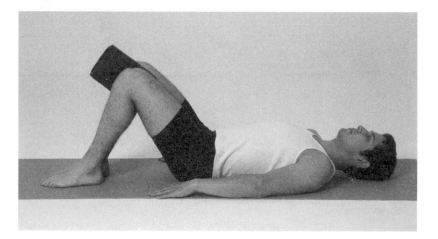

2. As you breathe out, draw your navel to your spine and squeeze the cushion with your knees, taking care not to let your back arch or tension creep into your back, shoulders or neck. Your knees shoud be the only part of your body that are moving.

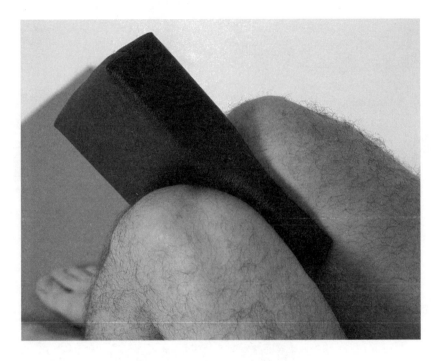

3. Breathe in to release. Repeat up to 10 times.

Part Four

8

Manipulative
Treatments

This final part of the book examines other therapies and lifestyle considerations that complement Pilates technique in helping to maintain a fit, strong and relaxed back. Each one works in its own unique way, whether by remedying an existing back problem, strengthening the whole system, or by overcoming the underlying stress that can cause or increase muscle tension.

Some of the therapies suggested here – massage, physiotherapy, osteopathy, for instance – obviously require you to visit a qualified practitioner (see the Resources chapter beginning on page 229 for recommended professional bodies). Others, however, are very much under your own control. These include simple hydrotherapy (page 203) or breathing techniques (page 221) and – one of the most important elements – your diet. A nutritious diet with a plentiful supply of important vitamins and minerals will help to keep your back healthy. On the other side of the coin, people who smoke suffer more disability through back pain than people who don't.

Not all of the therapies in this section may be appropriate for you, but some almost certainly will be of help with your back problem. Others are simply such a pleasant way of spending an hour that you might want to make them a habit for sheer self-indulgence.

Osteopathy and Chiropractic

These two manipulative therapies are closely related, both working principally on the musculo-skeletal system – the bones, joints, muscles, ligaments and connective tissues. They aim to diagnose and treat problems that occur because of injury, stress or disease, and to enable the musculo-skeletal system to work as efficiently as possible, allowing the body to restore itself to normal function. They are particularly valuable for back pain, sports injuries, neck tension, headaches (with a physical cause), arthritis and rheumatism. The two therapies have more in common than they differ, and individual therapists from one system often incorporate techniques from the other. As a very rough rule of thumb, though, a chiropractor manipulates directly over a joint, while an osteopath uses more leverage near to, but not over, the joint.

OSTEOPATHY

Dr Andrew Taylor Still (1828–1917) became the founder of osteopathy in the latter years of the 19th century. He practised medicine in Kirksville, Missouri but, though well versed in the orthodox medicine of the time, he became powerfully aware of its limitations when three of his young sons died of meningitis.

He strongly believed that doctors should find the means to stimulate the body's own healing mechanisms and to remove any obstacles to that process, rather than merely to try to suppress a particular disease or its symptoms. He based his approach on the principle that the body was able to heal itself or function well when it was structurally sound. Any structural abnormality he referred to as an 'osteopathic lesion' and this, he believed, would have to be removed for smooth functioning of all the systems of the body.

His breakthrough came during an epidemic of dysentery in 1874 when he successfully treated 18 cases by relieving muscular spasm in the back and restoring mobility to the joints. This confirmed his belief that the spine was the key to health, as it houses the spinal cord, the link between brain and body. This belief is still central to osteopathy, though it concerns itself too with the other organs and systems of the body. Dr Still himself was an early proponent of a holistic approach to health, seeing the physical, spiritual and mental as inextricably linked. He founded the first school of osteopathy in 1892. More schools followed rapidly, first in the US, then in the UK and Europe.

It is the nature of osteopathy to treat not just a localized problem or injury, but the overall health and condition of the patient. Given this approach, osteopaths are often able to identify and correct not only the injury itself, but other underlying problems which, if left untreated, may emerge in later life. This holistic approach to diagnosis and treatment is regarded as one of the most valuable aspects of osteopathy.

A caring approach and attention to the individual is considered particularly important in osteopathy, and you can expect a lengthy initial consultation. This may include taking a full and detailed medical history, visual observation of how you lie down, stand, sit and move, and various tests (blood pressure, testing reflexes, perhaps arranging X-rays). It will certainly also include the osteopath manually checking your joints, tissues, muscles and skin tone. It may at this point become clear to the osteopath that osteopathy is not, in fact, the answer, in which case your therapist will advise medical or complementary treatment elsewhere.

If you go ahead with osteopathic treatment, the osteopath will use one of three main techniques, according to your specific problem:

1. Soft tissue work uses stretching, rolling and kneading movements to stimulate circulation and relax the muscles and ligaments. This may be very gentle and subtle, or may entail increasing pressure.

2   Articulation is the mobilizing of your joints through their range of movement. This not only loosens tight joints, it affects related ligaments and muscles, too.

3. Manipulation is the thrust by which an osteopath returns a joint to its correct position. This can be a sudden movement (you may be asked to help by breathing in or out at the appropriate moment) or more indirect and subtle.

Treatments generally last 20 to 30 minutes and, in some cases, one session will be sufficient. It is more usual, though, to take a course of treatments, particularly if your condition is deep-seated or if you have had it for a long time. The treatment should not be painful – though there may be some discomfort at times. Many patients simply find it relaxing, and some even fall asleep while the osteopath works. After treatment your osteopath may give you advice on how to maintain your health with remedial exercises to adjust posture, or information on diet and lifestyle.

CHIROPRACTIC

Chiropractic was introduced at the end of the 19th century by the American healer David Daniel Palmer. He focused on spinal manipulation as a means of curing not only musculo-skeletal conditions but also problems as diverse as heart disease and loss of hearing. His philosophy was that displaced vertebrae in the spine restrict the spinal nerves and this, in turn, prevents the body's proper flow of energy.

Chiropractic has developed over the last century and practitioners now use direct pressure on the spine and joints in a form of manipulation known simply as 'adjustment'. By squeezing, pulling or twisting the limbs, torso or head, the chiropractor readjusts the spinal column to place the vertebrae in the correct position. As well as treating back problems and relieving back pain, chiropractors also do preventative work, looking for misalignments and correcting them before they become a problem or injury.

The vast majority of chiropractic patients have back problems – joint problems, strains and back pain being the most common. When you visit a chiropractor, he or she will take a detailed case history, give you a complete physical examination and may take various tests, such as blood pressure, blood and urine analysis, X-rays or other diagnostic procedures. This will establish whether chiropractic is the right treatment for you.

If you decide to go ahead, the treatment itself will be manipulation directly over your spine or affected joints. Sometimes you may hear a sound, as if a joint is being popped back into its proper place, though the noise is actually caused by the movement of bubbles of nitrogen around the joint. The therapist may also massage the related muscles and give you advice on exercises to do at home.

Massage

There are many kinds of massage, but it may be helpful when considering how they can help back problems to divide them into two categories – remedial and relaxing. All massage works on the muscles and soft tissues.

REMEDIAL MASSAGE

As its name implies, this addresses a specific injury or ailment. It is particularly effective with joint problems, chronic muscular stiffness, especially in the lumbar region, the shoulders and neck, and stress-related conditions resulting in muscle tension. The masseur works on the problem muscles, stimulating the oxygen and blood supply to them, and so increasing the shedding of toxins that build up around tensed muscles, causing stiffness and pain. The therapist will often give advice on posture and exercise in order to help you avoid further problems. Remedial massage therapists can be found in most sports centres, gyms and leisure centres. Several sessions may be needed for the best results.

RELAXING MASSAGE

Massage for relaxation usually entails a whole-body massage. There are many different kinds of relaxing massage, but they all affect the mind as well as the body, as touch has the power to release not only tense muscles but mental stress and emotional tension, too. As tense muscles are often a direct result of emotional stress, relaxing massage works on several levels at once.

SWEDISH MASSAGE

This is a widely available form of often vigorous massage that uses a variety of strokes. These include hacking (a chopping movement with the sides of the hands), *effleurage* (a stroking movement), *petrissage* (squeezing the soft tissue against the bone), kneading (squeezing the soft tissue independently) and cupping (a quick movement cupping the hand to form a vacuum).

AROMATHERAPY MASSAGE

Another very popular form of massage, aromatherapy massage uses many of the same strokes as Swedish massage, but usually less vigorously. Most importantly, it uses essential oils, diluted in a carrier oil, that are absorbed through the skin and act on the sense of smell. Specific oils can be used to enhance the effect of relaxation, such as lavender, neroli (orange blossom), rose, jasmine and ylang-ylang.

THAI MASSAGE

For this massage, you are usually given loose pyjamas to wear as there is no direct contact with the skin. Thai massage is a combination of massage strokes and manipulation in which the therapist can use his or her elbows, feet and knees as well as hands. It can entail very strong pressure indeed, but is often wonderfully releasing.

SHIATSU

Shiatsu is a part of traditional Eastern medicine and uses the same principles as acupuncture in facilitating the flow of *chi*, or energy, through the body in a series of pathways or meridians. According to this philosophy, when the flow of chi is blocked, pain and ailments result. The massage usually takes place on a mat on the floor, rather than a massage table, and you remain clothed. As with Thai massage, the therapist can use his or her feet, knees and elbows as well as hands, sometimes with a strong pressure.

AYURVEDIC MASSAGE

This massage is a part of the ancient Indian healthcare system of Ayurveda. It comprises a whole range of massages, the two most common being *Abhyanga* and *Shirodhara*.

Abhyanga massage entails the use of warmed sesame oil and is administered by two masseurs at the same time, working in tandem on both sides of the body. Mostly, the strokes are long and firm and those parts of the body not being massaged are covered in hot towels.

In *Shirodhara*, a stream of sesame oil is drizzled onto the forehead from a dish with a hole pierced in it. The oil begins on the centre of the forehead and moves slowly from side to side, for in all about 20 minutes.

The two treatments are often given together to achieve total relaxation of body and mind.

Physiotherapy

Physiotherapy is a healthcare profession concerned with human function and movement. Every year, Britain's 40,000 chartered physiotherapists help millions of people manage the effects of illness, accidents, disability and the stresses and strains of everyday life. They use a broad range of techniques to help muscle and joints work to their full potential. Physiotherapy can help repair damage by optimizing the healing process and reducing pain and stiffness.

Physiotherapists are experts in movement, from the way we move our backs or limbs, to the way we breathe. The prime purpose of physiotherapy is to restore function, activity and independence, prevent injury or illness, by using manual techniques and providing information and advice on healthy lifestyles. Physiotherapists work with both adults and children and offer a multi-faceted approach to the management of a wide range of conditions.

The physiotherapy assessment is detailed and involves a holistic approach to the presenting problem. The aim is then to explain, i) the pathology of the condition to the client, ii) the linkage between the mind and the body, iii) the plan of action in agreement with the client.

Banish Back Pain the Pilates Way

It is vitally important that a thorough explanation is given. Compliance will be so much greater.

One aim is to improve posture and try to achieve perfect alignment of all joints, so that tissues will function in their rightful position. All tissues require oxygen to survive and so manual techniques are used both to achieve the best oxygen flow to all tissues, and to assist in restoring the alignment of the joints.

The treatments used include: manipulation and mobilization of soft tissues and joints, mobilization of neural tissue, acupuncture, electrotherapy, including ultrasound and interferential, reflextherapy, hydrotherapy and exercises in water and exercise rehabilitation. All physiotherapists are experienced in understanding muscle imbalance. With this awareness, many physiotherapists are trained in Pilates rehabilitation.

Physiotherapists aim to resolve the presenting condition. They also aim to advise on prevention of other conditions developing, and frequently pick up on areas which may lead to problems later. Physiotherapy can help with virtually any condition that affects muscles, joints or nerves. Common problems that can be helped by physiotherapists include:

Manipulative Treatments

painful conditions such as arthritis, back and neck pain (including whiplash), problems affecting children (including cerebral palsy), pregnancy related symptoms such as back pain and stress incontinence, upper limb work related problems, also known as repetitive strain injury (RSI), asthma and other breathing difficulties, sports injuries, strokes and other neurological problems, and symptoms of stress and anxiety.

CHOOSING A PHYSIOTHERAPIST

Chartered physiotherapists can be found in a variety of settings – hospitals, health centres, GP practices, industry, schools, leisure centres. Some will visit you in the NHS, others have their own practices. Your GP can refer you to your local physiotherapy service. Alternatively, you can visit a chartered physiotherapist privately. Contact names and numbers can be found in directories such as Yellow Pages or you can contact the Organisation of Chartered Physiotherapists in Private Practice on 01702 392 124.

When choosing a private physiotherapist make sure they have at least one of the following sets of initials after their name: MCSP (Member of the Chartered Society of Physiotherapy) or SRP (State Registered Physiotherapist). This will guarantee that they are properly qualified (usually after a three-to-four-year degree course); governed by a professional code of conduct; and covered by professional liability insurance.

Water Treatments

Because water supports your weight, it can be a very good medium in which to increase mobility and ease tension. You can use water for this purpose in a number of ways. First, you can exercise in it, whether by swimming or by doing specific exercises to ease a back problem. Secondly, you can try out one of the several water-based spa therapies that are becoming increasingly widely available. And finally, there are numerous home treatments that will help to relax and release tense or immobile muscles and joints.

THE BENEFITS OF SWIMMING

Swimming is one of the most beneficial forms of aerobic exercise, as well as one of the safest. It is not a high-impact activity like running, so many people who have sustained injuries – especially back and joint injuries – can swim safely without fear of further damage. It is a particularly beneficial form of exercise for anyone with stiff joints, too – whether from general lack of exercise or due to a specific condition, such as arthritis – because it will often loosen up the problem areas without the risk of jerky, and hence potentially damaging, movements. For this very reason, swimming is probably the best form of exercise for the elderly, who are particularly likely to suffer from joint problems.

For anyone who is overweight, swimming is a very good way to start an exercise programme, and indeed to lose weight. Exercising on dry land can be particularly hazardous for anyone who is overweight, because most land exercise is, by definition, weight-bearing, and the extra weight becomes an additional strain on the joints, muscles and ligaments, predisposing them to injury. Swimming, on the other hand, reduces these risks dramatically.

Of course, anyone overweight is also putting an extra strain on the heart when exercising, so some caution must be used, especially if you are starting to exercise after a long break. Build up gradually and take it slowly at first. If you are seriously overweight, get medical advice before you start.

Some swimming strokes are going to be safer than others if you have back problems. The breast stroke is beneficial if your back is generally trouble free, but it is not recommended for anyone with neck, lumbar or other back problems, or for pregnant women. The crawl is excellent aerobic exercise, good for toning arm muscles and for releasing stiff shoulder joints. The gentlest stroke, if you have had back problems recently, is the back stroke. It releases and mobilizes the shoulder joints, and is also the best stroke for pregnant women.

Manipulative Treatments   **199**

WATER AEROBICS

Water aerobics is, quite simply, exercising in water. It draws both on rehabilitative hydrotherapy techniques and ordinary land-based forms of aerobic exercise. For the same reasons as swimming, it is a good way to get fit without risk of injury. And, because you can also use the resistance of water almost as you would use weights or machines, it is excellent for targeting particular areas of the body.

There are water aerobics classes available at most swimming pools and health clubs. As with any form of exercise, it is always better to have a teacher supervising you, at least to start with. However, here are some simple water aerobics movements for specific results or to relieve particular problems.

Arm Lunges

This exercises increases mobility in the neck, shoulders and the lower back, as well as simultaneously toning the arms.

1. Stand in the pool with the water at shoulder level, feet hip-width apart, your hands on your hips.

2. Breathe in and, as you breathe out, draw your navel to your spine

and take your right arm to shoulder height and reach across your body, bending your left leg as you do so and pushing the water away.

3. Repeat, alternating sides, 10 times.

Squats

Squats mobilize your spine at the same time as toning your legs and buttocks. Remember to keep your navel drawn to your spine throughout.

1. Stand at the side of the pool, holding onto the ledge with both hands, your legs hip-width apart with the water chest-high. Place your feet so that your knees are pointing slightly outwards, keeping your feet and knees in line.

2. Breathe in and, as you breathe out, draw your navel to your spine and bend your knees so that the tail of your spine drops straight down towards the bottom of the pool – no arching in the lower spine. Hold for a count of 10, then come up. Repeat up to 10 times.

Scissors

This exercise tones the abdominal muscles – but try to keep the rest of your body still.

1. Stretch out on top of the water, facing downwards and holding on to the ledge.

2. Breathe in and, as you breathe out, draw your navel to your spine. Holding your abdominal muscles in strongly and keeping your legs underwater, scissor your legs up and down as if you were taking giant-sized straight-legged steps.

Shoulder Circles

This exercise increases mobility in the neck and shoulders. It is essentially the same as the exercise on page 84, but many people find it easier to relax when in the water.

1. Stand in the pool with your feet slightly apart, the water up to your neck.

2. Breathe in and, as you breathe out, draw your navel to your spine and slowly circle your shoulders, taking them forwards, upwards and back 10 times.

3. Then reverse the movement for another 10 circles.

Leg Swings

This exercise improves mobility in the hip joints and the lower back generally. It also tones the legs. If you feel a strain in your back at any time, stop immediately.

1. Stand at the side of the pool with good posture, the feet hip-width apart and one hand resting on the edge.

2. Breathe in and, as you breathe out, take your right leg out in front of you, keeping the knee facing forwards and your leg straight. Swing the leg in front and then behind you 10 times.

3. Turn and repeat on the other leg.

TAKING THE HEAT

As we have already seen, heat is an excellent way of relaxing tense muscles, including muscle spasms. In Part Two advice was given on topical heat applications, but a heated environment can also be very beneficial.

Steam baths are a very widespread form of heat treatment and come in many forms. The communal steam room is becoming increasingly popular and can be found in most health clubs and spas. There are also individual steam baths or cabinets, in which your head remains outside the cabinet – and so stays cooler than the rest of your body – and which some people find more comfortable than being in a steam room.

Saunas are another popular form of heat treatment. While the heat of a sauna is dry, the dry heat can be alternated with cool or cold showers or plunge-pools. This combination can stimulate the whole system. As with steam baths, saunas relax and promote toxin elimination through sweating.

With both steam baths and saunas, there are a few precautions to remember. Most importantly, don't stay in too long – 20 minutes is plenty, less if you're not used to it, and you should come out if you feel dizzy or uncomfortable. Lie down and relax as much as possible while you are in the sauna or steam room, and always rest afterwards to give your body time to return to its normal temperature and functioning. Don't eat within an hour before or after a sauna or steam bath, but drink plenty of water. Wear as little as possible and always take off any jewellery – the metal will heat up rapidly and burn you.

WATER MASSAGE

There are a number of water treatments that incorporate massage to produce a deep relaxation of both body and mind and, because the water supports your weight, your back can relax in a way that is impossible when lying on an ordinary massage table. Water massages are sometimes mechanical or they can be performed by a therapist.

HYDROTHERAPY BATHS

Being submerged in water, especially warm water, is in itself relaxing. Heat makes the muscles relax and the joints soften, as well as bringing a state of tranquillity to the mind. The gentle massage of water in the form of underwater jets helps relieve stiffness and sprains, as well as being pleasantly relaxing and improving the circulation. Jacuzzis are the most widespread form of these underwater jet massages, but hydrotherapy baths are also on the increase.

Hydrotherapy baths have been used therapeutically in many European countries for over a century, as a part of the regular annual 'cure' that was taken annually. The cure would act as a general detoxification – long before it became a popular concept in the 1990s – addressing not only diet, but also skin, respiratory and joint problems, in particular.

The baths themselves are shaped like an ordinary bath but incorporate various forms of water massage methods that can alternate during treatment. One is a general water-jet massage, much like that of a jacuzzi, although as you are lying down it is even more relaxing. The other is a more intense massage that begins at the feet and works its way slowly up the entire length of the body. One of the most relaxing baths I've experienced was in the north Italian spa town of Salsomaggiore, where they used the disarmingly simple method of a hose with an extremely powerful jet in a very deep bath. The effect was enhanced by using the local heavily mineralized water (see page 205 for more on this). After 20 minutes I was left feeling relaxed to the point of jelly-like bones!

MASSAGE ON WATER

A comparatively recent innovation is the hydrotherm spa massage system. Essentially, it consists of being massaged on a giant hot-water bottle – one of those ideas that is so simple you can't understand how nobody came up with it before. It is particularly helpful for anyone who has recently suffered an attack of acute back pain or has on-going chronic back pain, as the heat helps any muscles that are in spasm to relax.

The hydrotherm unit is the length of your torso, reaching up as far as your neck, with your head resting on a separate, unheated pillow for comfort. You lie on your back and allow the heat to penetrate, soothing any aches and pains and making the muscles relax. The therapist then gives you a back massage that is made doubly effective because of the heat. The first time I tried it, it felt a little strange, because the water was moving beneath me constantly. However, after a few minutes I relaxed into the soothing feeling of being gently rocked on water. It is, incidentally, a boon for pregnant women who often suffer from backache but, for obvious reasons, can't have a normal massage where they would lie on their fronts. It is also a good way to have a massage if you are underweight, fragile or elderly.

MASSAGE IN WATER

This is another comparatively new – and, sadly, as yet rare – form of massage, in which the therapist gets into the water with you. The water itself is heavily salinated, either with Epsom Salts, as in a floatation tank (see page 206) or with highly mineralized water, which has the same supportive effect. I tried it at Le Meridien Spa in Cyprus, where they have one of the most complete – and beautiful – hydrotherapy spas, and where they use Dead Sea mineral salts to keep you afloat.

As you get into the warm water, you put on an eye mask to protect your eyes from the salts – if the water were to get into your eyes it would sting. However, a side-effect of wearing the eye mask, combined with the loss of hearing because your ears are underwater, means that your paramount sense throughout is touch – and this makes the massage more powerful still. The therapist then helps you into position – essentially, you simply float on top of the buoyant water, the therapist simultaneously supporting and manipulating different parts of your body.

The massage is more manipulation than the usual massage, and it is especially good for locked joints, the arms and legs being rotated to free up the shoulder and hip joints. The back is also mobilized significantly, both with twisting movements and sideways stretches. The warmth of the water, the minerals and the sensation of weightlessness make this an exceptionally relaxing and releasing massage.

FLOATATION

The aim of floating, as has already been touched on, is to relax both mind and body, though initially it may seem an odd sort of therapy. Before I tried it, I thought it would be too claustrophobic to be relaxing, as it often takes place inside a covered tank. In fact, after about 15 minutes I found myself totally at ease in my watery environment, turned out the lights and floated contentedly for the rest of my hour.

Unless you happen to be an astronaut, floating is the only time your body is going to be free of the forces of gravity, and this is in itself quite an extraordinary feeling. The combination of weightlessness and the absence of external stimuli enables the body to relax deeply – I experienced an almost instant release of tension in the small of my back that I didn't even know I had. This is a very common reaction to floating, and back sufferers generally report it to be particularly beneficial. The water is at body temperature and your head is supported on an inflated cushion so that the salinated water does not sting your eyes. The benefits, though, are believed to be more than just physical.

According to the floatation research, external stimuli – gravity, temperature, touch, sight, sound – account for 90 per cent of normal neuro-muscular activity. When they are absent, even for an hour, the brain and the rest of the nervous system can achieve a state that is not only relaxing but, it is believed, rebalancing. Activity in the left, logical side of the brain is reduced and activity in the right, creative side increases. Adherents of floating believe that this is one of the few times your brain is in a state of harmony and that this helps you tap into a huge, previously unavailable source of creativity, imagination and problem-solving.

Physical Effects of Floating

Because floating causes the muscles to relax so profoundly and the body to release endorphins (your body's own painkillers), floating is a powerful aid to pain relief and very helpful during an attack of back pain (providing you are helped in and out of the tank). By relieving the stresses of gravity, it takes the weight off strained bones, joints and muscles, as well as increasing the efficiency of the blood circulation, and this in turn speeds up recovery after injury or physical exercise. What normally takes a long period of time – say, several days to recover after running a marathon – can be compressed into a matter of hours. This has made floating popular among professional sportsmen and – women.

Like other forms of profound relaxation, floating lowers blood pressure and heart rate. And, because of the salts in the water, it is even beneficial to the skin.

In the tank

Seven hundred pounds of Epsom Salts are added to 170 gallons of water; the salts are what make you so buoyant and give the water its silky feel. Within the tank the water level is around 10 inches deep and the water itself is heated to 93.5 degrees, which is skin temperature. There is a light within the tank and you can, of course, leave this on if you wish. I had thought I would, especially after I closed the tank doors so that I was sealed inside. However, there is quite a lot of space above you when you are in the tank and, in the event, the environment felt so relaxing, I floated in the dark.

Music is often played for the first 10 minutes while you relax, but for most of the time that you are floating, you are surrounded only by silence. There is also evidence that audio-tape programmes for weight loss or overcoming addictions such as smoking can be incorporated in the treatment to great effect.

THALASSOTHERAPY

Thalassotherapy is a form of hydrotherapy that uses sea water or other sea substances – notably minerals, seaweed and/or mud extracted from the sea and sand. The spa at Le Meridien in Cyprus is a particularly good example of the 'new' popularity of thalassotherapy, with an extensive range of treatments using water and sea treatments and products. Rosmoney Spa in Ireland is another 'new' thalassotherapy spa, using the local seaweed and sea minerals, as well as drawing on the water from the Atlantic. Traditionally, thalassotherapy is particularly popular in France, Germany, Italy, Russia and, most famously of all, around the Dead Sea.

Thalassotherapy is beneficial for a number of back problems, especially muscle and joint problems, rheumatism and arthritis. It is, incidentally, also of benefit for respiratory, circulatory and skin disorders. The Dead Sea itself is the mother of all floatation tanks. You walk in and simply get pushed up to the surface by the buoyancy of the water. It can be as painful for the eyes or any cuts or grazes as a floatation tank with Epsom Salts, but its efficacy with joint and muscular problems is renowned.

As well as floating in the Dead Sea itself, you can experience its benefits in the Zara Spa in Jordan on the banks of the Sea. Here, there are large indoor and outdoor heated or cool pools of cleansed Dead Sea water in various strengths, so you can move from one to another to get the traditional hydrotherapy benefits of temperature changes. The mud and salts from the sea are also used by therapists in the form of scrubs and body wraps, combined with heating treatments and 'dry floatation', where your massage table turns into a bath of heated sea water and you float on top in your body wrap.

Other forms of thalassotherapy use the products of different seas. Seaweed can be used in its natural form (as at Rosmoney Spa in Ireland) in the bath, rather like a loofah, its oils massage into your skin. At Rosmoney, all the treatments use water from the Atlantic, cleansed but still in a highly mineralized state, and even swimming in the sea-water pool benefits joint and muscle problems. As a more general boost to health, sea water is believed to encourage detoxification and increase immunity, stimulate circulation of blood and lymph, soothe and help tone muscles and improve skin tone.

THERAPEUTIC BATHS

There are a number of spa baths that work equally well in the home and are very easy to set up. The extra ingredients these particular baths use, if any, are cheap and easily available, yet the results can be very beneficial indeed.

Ordinary baths of various temperatures can be very effective for particular conditions. A hot bath, for instance, because it encourages blood flow to the part of the body that is submerged, can be very soothing for lower back pain. Warm baths are very good for the release of tension in the body, and work well if you have trouble sleeping caused by chronic back pain. In this case, try a full bath of tepid water, staying in it for up to 30 minutes, just before you go to bed.

For a more heating bath, and very helpful for releasing muscle spasm, you can add Epsom Salts. This may sound very old-fashioned, but it is one of the most relaxing baths you can find. The magnesium in the Epsom Salts warms and soothes the body, which helps the joints and muscles unwind. It's more than just warming, though. In fact, you can expect to get very hot indeed and, as your temperature rises, not only do your joints and muscles relax, you will sweat out toxins rapidly. Epsom Salts usually come in 2-kg (4-lb) packs, and you just throw the lot into the bath. It takes quite a lot of stirring to mix it all in, but it is important that they have dissolved thoroughly before you get in.

Epsom Salts are available at pharmacists and health-food shops. If you have difficulty tracking them down, though, you can substitute herbs and spices – ginger, sage and cayenne pepper have a similar effect in terms of raising the temperature!

Whatever you are using as your heating agent, lie in the bath for at least 15 minutes. You can expect to sweat copiously – but this is all just a natural part of the process. You can increase the heating effect by massaging your body with a loofah or bath mitt.

MOOR AND MUD

Mud may not be one of the most glamorous forms of treatment in the world, but it is one of the oldest. Mud packs were used by the ancient Egyptians and Romans for various ailments and as beauty treatments, and similar treatments have always been available at hydrotherapy spas, most notably in Europe. Therapeutic mud often comes from areas around mineral springs; the high mineral content of the mud is often put forward as one of the main reasons for its curative powers.

One of the most famous sources of therapeutic mud is the Neydharting Moor, about 60 kilometres from Salzburg in Austria. Archaeological finds there have shown that it was in use from as early as 800BC by the Celts, who were followed, later, by the Romans. There is a thriving clinic at Neydharting today, which is so renowned within Europe that there is a very long waiting list to get in.

Known just as 'Moor' or 'Moor-Life', the mud has been investigated and analysed by over 500 scientists and declared unique. Because the 20,000-year-old glacial valley basin in which it lies was first a lake and then a moor, where the waters have never been drained away, it has retained all of its organic, mineral and trace elements. It is especially rich in decomposed plant life: of over 1,000 plant deposits – flowering herbs, seeds, leaves, flowers, tubers, fruits roots and grasses – some 300 of them have recognized medical properties. Medical evidence shows that the Moor's properties are both anti-inflammatory and astringent, making it particularly useful for back problems related to rheumatism and arthritis.

HOME TREATMENTS

There are many therapists who use Moor products besides those at the clinic in Austria, and you can also buy products to use at home. The most useful for back sufferers is the Moor bath, which comes in a large can that looks like a motor oil container. It does look exactly like mud, and you need to mix it in well with the water of your bath or it will form little globules and not be nearly as effective. The water should be warm, not hot, and you should stay in for at least half an hour, topping up with warm water as necessary. This is not a bath to wash in – so don't use any soaps or shampoos. If you want to do that, have a shower first and then let yourself soak in the mud bath. If possible, have a Moor bath late at night and go to bed straight away – it is a very relaxing bath and you usually sleep particularly well after it.

Dead Sea products are also available for home use. The mineral-rich mud is 'mined' and purified, then packaged – either still in its mud form or as extracted mineral salts. It contains an extraordinary range of minerals, principally potassium, which helps regulate the body's water balance, and bromine, sulphur and iodine, which stimulate cell rejuvenation and repair while promoting an increase in the blood supply to the skin. In addition, there are small quantities of other minerals – 25 in all – including significant quantities of zinc and copper, the minerals often found lacking in people with arthritis. Dead Sea products are particularly effective at reducing inflammation and swelling and increasing mobility.

These products are widely available, and the most potent for therapeutic use are the Dead Sea bath salts, which should be used in exactly the same way as the Moor mud bath, again ideally last thing at night.

Many seaweed products are also available for home use. You can buy organic seaweed fresh in health-food stores, or buy a ready-made powder. Seaweed itself is packed with vital nutrients – minerals and vitamins, enzymes and amino acids – which are absorbed through the skin while you bathe. As with all of the other therapeutic baths, this is not one to wash in. If you want to, shower first, then just lie in the warm – not hot – seaweed water for at least half an hour, topping up the warm water as necessary. Pat yourself gently to dry, then rest for at least half an hour, or take the bath last thing at night and go straight to bed.

AROMATHERAPY BATHS

One of the most appealing water treatments is bathing with aromatherapy oils. Not only are you immersed in warm water, the oil has very beneficial effects on your skin, as it relaxes tense joints and muscles and you are surrounded by the loveliest scents. A number of oils are very effective in relaxing both body and mind, especially when used in the bath. Last thing at night, an aromatherapy bath will relax tense muscles and prepare you for a restful sleep, slowing down your mind and relaxing your body at the end of the day.

Fill the bath with water – it shouldn't be too hot or the oil will simply evaporate – and, when it is ready, add 5 to 10 drops of your chosen oil to the water and swish around so that it is mixed in well. Stay in the bath for at least 20 minutes and relax. When you come out of the bath, wrap yourself in a big, warm towel, but don't dry yourself vigorously. Pat gently with the towel or sit wrapped up in it until it absorbs the water on your body. This way, you keep a little of the oil on your skin. Put on a dressing gown or pyjamas, or get into bed straight away to stay warm and relaxed.

Relaxing Oils

For a relaxing bath that will release tense muscles and promote a deep, restful sleep, choose one of the following oils.

- Lavender is one of the most gentle oils. It is a soporific and it also relieves headaches and physical and mental stress. If you have trouble sleeping, you can also put a drop or two on your pillow, or apply it very gently to your temples.
- Neroli is extracted from the blossom of the orange tree and has a quite sensational smell. It lifts the spirits, as well as being generally calming, and is particularly beneficial for mature skin.
- Sandalwood has a warm, woody fragrance and is an anti-depressant as well as a soporific. Men often find this more appealing than floral scents and it is used in many men's toiletries.

Diet and Nutrition

While extensive advice on diet is beyond the scope of this book, there are a few guidelines to bear in mind on healthy eating. Healthy eating supports all of the body's systems, enhancing its performance generally and reducing its susceptibility to infection, ailments and degenerative diseases.

One of the most important factors when considering diet in relation to back problems is weight. Being overweight is much more likely to lead to back and joint problems simply because carrying the extra weight puts so much more strain on the body. Resulting problems are most likely to occur in the lower back, where the strain is felt most.

If you are overweight, it is much better to try to lose the excess by following a balanced, healthy diet than by crash-dieting, which will usually result in nutritional imbalance. Aim for a large proportion of fresh fruit and vegetables in your diet – regard the five daily portions recommended by the World Health Organization as the minimum. Protein should account for 10–15 per cent of your diet, choosing oily fish, such as tuna and sardines, rather than red meat and eggs. Dairy produce can be eaten in moderation, but choose low-fat versions whenever possible. Avoid fats, especially saturated fats (those found in junk food, butter, farmed meat and full-fat dairy produce). Fats are often combined with sugars in cakes, pastry and biscuits. Sugars should be avoided, too. Starchy foods used to be regarded as the ones that made you overweight, but in fact they can help to control weight, being very satisfying yet low in fat. Starchy foods include cereals such as wheat, oats, barley and rice, and some vegetables, such as potatoes.

There are also some specific nutrients that contribute to back health:

ANTI-OXIDANTS

The vitamins A, C and E, together with the minerals zinc and selenium, are known as anti-oxidants. Many of the B-complex vitamins and certain amino acids have anti-oxidant properties, too. They can protect us not only against minor infections, but also lower the risk of serious degenerative diseases, as well as the conditions that come with premature ageing. They work by acting as scavengers for free radicals, electrochemically unbalanced molecules that are generated within our bodies by, among other things, pollution, cigarettes, pesticides, drugs, certain foods, overeating and stress. Free radicals are responsible at a cellular level for many of the things that go wrong with the body. Anti-oxidant nutrients also promote the growth of strong bones, muscles and connective tissues. Good sources of anti-oxidants include fresh fruits and vegetables (especially green, leafy vegetables), nuts and seeds (sunflower, pumpkin and sesame seeds, hazelnuts, chestnuts, brazil nuts, almonds), beans and lentils, oily fish and game.

CALCIUM

This is the basic mineral in bones and teeth. It is necessary to replace it constantly, but particularly after the menopause when a lack of calcium can result in osteoporosis. Milk has high levels of calcium and also of vitamin D, which enhances the body's ability to absorb calcium. Choose low-fat options, especially yoghurt. Other foods with calcium include almonds, apples and pears, beans and lentils, vegetables (including cabbage, carrots, spinach, watercress), oats, soya and nuts (cashews, walnuts).

MAGNESIUM, PHOSPHORUS AND SILICON

These three minerals are all important for bone health. Good sources include green leafy vegetables, beans and lentils, berries, apples and pears, seaweed and sea vegetables, soya, sweet potatoes, oats and beetroot.

WATER

While you can't classify water strictly as a food, it is essential to life and the smooth functioning of every part and system of the body. Without enough water, body and mind become sluggish and less efficient. Our bodies are – or should be – at least 70 per cent water. However, because we lose water all the time – through urination, every time we breathe

out, and a staggering 1 litre (1¾ pints) per day through the skin alone –
to replenish the necessary levels we should drink a minimum of 2 litres,
or about 8 glasses, every day. Filtered or bottled water is best, herbal
teas and juices are also good. However, tea, coffee and alcohol, while
acceptable in moderation, in excess dehydrate the body.

Breathing and Meditation Techniques

There are various ways in which the breath can be used to relax the
body and even help with pain control. If your back pain is keeping you
awake, breathing techniques are particularly useful in treating insomnia
and settling the mind, facilitating a deeper and easier sleep. These
techniques are beneficial, too, as a means of stress-relief throughout the
day, in particular if you are under a lot of pressure at work or at home
and you feel tension building up, especially in your shoulders and neck.

PRANAYAMA

This breathing technique is a yoga exercise. *Prana* is the flow of energy
through the body and a means of eliminating blockages that cause pain
and tension. *Pranayama*, as its name suggests, is closely linked to the

concept of prana. It improves oxygen intake and circulation, and increases the flow of oxygen to every cell in the body. It is a method of obtaining deep relaxation and can be used at times of stress to dispel tension, when breathing typically becomes fast and shallow.

1. Sit on a chair that supports your spine so that you feel comfortable and relaxed. If you prefer, you can kneel or sit cross-legged on the floor, but your back must be as straight as possible and held without tension. Choose whichever position is most comfortable for you – this will support your pranayama best.

2. Close your eyes and breathe in. With your left hand resting in your lap, lift your right hand up to be level with your face and, using your thumb, close your right nostril.

3. Exhale through your left nostril, slowly and easily. Then breathe in, slowly and easily again.

4. Now close off your left nostril with the middle finger of your right hand. Exhale, then take your thumb away from your right nostril and inhale slowly.

5. Continue, alternating nostrils, for about 5 minutes. Your breathing should be as natural as possible, not exaggerated, though it may be a little slower and deeper than usual.

6. After 5 minutes, sit quietly with your eyes closed and breathe normally for a few minutes.

ABDOMINAL BREATHING

This exercise is very relaxing if you try to focus completely on what your breath is doing, following it with your mind as it travels through your body.

1. Lie in the Corpse pose (see page 56) on a blanket on the floor, covering yourself with another blanket if you feel cold. Your spine should be in one long line, continuing up through your neck to the top of your head. Let your feet and legs roll out so they are relaxed, and place your arms a little way from your sides, palms up. Check through your body for signs of tension and release as much as you can.

2. Place one hand on your abdomen and the other on your chest. Feel your body move with your breath. If the hand on your chest moves

more than the one on your abdomen, your breath is only reaching a small proportion of your body.

3. On the next breath, exhale as fully as you can so that you push the air out from the bottom of your lungs. Now breathe in through your nose again for as long as you can until you feel your abdomen rise, not just your chest.

4. Inhaling and exhaling only through your nose, continue to take long, slow abdominal breaths for a few minutes.

5. Return to your normal breathing for a few minutes before getting up.

MEDITATION

Long-term stress, as we have seen, can be a contributing factor in muscle tension and back pain. Rather surprisingly – for a practice in which to the observer it appears that nothing much is happening – regular meditation has emerged as one of the most effective ways of achieving deep relaxation and stress-release.

A considerable body of clinical research – focusing principally on the most dramatic and measurable manifestations of stress, such as heart disease – has shown that meditation results in substantial reductions in high blood pressure and cholesterol levels. Other clinical tests have shown that the risk of much of the physical and mental deterioration associated with ageing is reduced considerably by regular meditation.

A SIMPLE MEDITATION

The main thing to remember when learning to meditate is that the intrusion of thoughts is inevitable. Do not try too hard – you are not supposed to be forcing your mind into concentrating on a particular image. In fact, you are trying to release yourself from conscious thought. When anything – thoughts, worries, ideas, lists of what you have to do when you stop meditating – enters your mind, observe its presence gently, make no judgement about the thought itself and, above all, do not become irritated with yourself for having it! Having recognized the thought, let it go and draw your focus back to your breath, word or the image on which you are meditating.

You need to be comfortable but alert to meditate. You should also avoid being disturbed. Take the phone off the hook, find a quiet spot, wear loose, comfortable clothing and take off your shoes. You don't have to sit cross-legged on the floor – though you can if this is comfortable for you. You do, though, need to sit with a straight back and stay still for 20 minutes, so find a chair with good back support in which to do your meditation.

Before you begin, take some slow, deep breaths and try to let go of any areas of tension. Scan your mind for immediate thoughts and worries, then leave them on one side for later so your mind is clear to meditate.

There are many meditation techniques. Here I've suggested three. Try them out to see which one suits you best – but give each one about 10 days before you decide whether to try another. When you have found a method you like, the most important thing is to practise it regularly. Try to make your meditation session the same time of day in the same place every day. When you've become adept, you will be able to meditate at any time and in all kinds of places – even when there is noise or other people around.

BREATHING MEDITATION

Close your eyes and count each breath. Inhale on one, exhale on two, inhale on three, and so on. The breath should be even and you can focus the counting on either the sensation of the air entering through your nose or the rise and fall of your abdomen. If you lose count – and you will! – start again at one.

MANTRA

This is the silent repetition of a word. It can be a word with significance for you, like 'peace', or one that has a resonant sound – the best-known being the 'Om' mantra (pronounced 'aum'). Your aim is to reach a stage where the sound and resonance fill your mind.

VISUALIZATION

This can take the form of a place or an object, real or imagined, that you look at with your mind's eye. You picture this in the greatest detail, focusing completely upon it. A place of great tranquillity has a particularly calming influence in this meditation.

After 20 minutes, let the focus of your meditation fade gently away, and bring your mind back to the present. Take some long, deep breaths and let your focus take in your body and how it is feeling, gradually becoming aware of your surroundings and the noises around you. Open your eyes, but remain sitting still for a few more minutes.

Resources

US
Professional Bodies

American Osteopathic Association
142 East Ohio Street
Chicago, Illinois 60611
+ 1 312 280 5800

American Naturopathic Association
1413 King Street, First Floor
Washington DC 20005
+ 1 202 682 7352

American Chiropractic Association
1701 Clarendon Boulevard
Arlington, Virginia 22209
+ 1 703 276 8800

American Physical Therapy Association
1111 North Fairfax Street
Alexandria, VA 22314–1488
www.apta.org
+ 1 703 684 2782

UK

The Pilates Room
69a Waldemar Avenue
Fulham, London
SW6 5LR
020 7736 0992
www.thepilatesroom.org.uk

Professional Bodies

British School of Osteopathy
275 Borough High Street
London SE1
020 7407 0222

*British Osteopathic and Naturopathic
College and Clinic*
6 Netherhall Gardens
London NW3
020 7435 7830

*London College of Osteopathic
Medicine*
8 Boston Place
London NW1
020 7262 1128

British Chiropractic Association
Blagrave House
17 Blagrave Street
Reading
Berkshire RG1 1QB
0118 9505950

National Back Pain Association
16 Elmtree Road
Teddington
Middlesex TW11 8ST

Chartered Society of Physiotherapy
14 Bedford Row
London WC1R 4ED
020 7306 6666

Spas

Details of the spas mentioned in this book offering treatments that can be beneficial for back problems:

Le Meridien
Limassol
Cyprus
+ 357 5 634222
www.lemeridien-cyprus.com
The best thalassotherapy spa in the eastern Mediterranean, with indoor and outdoor sea-water pools, underwater massage and full range of other massages

Zara Spa
Movenpick Resort and Spa
Sweimah
Jordan
+ 962 5356 1110
www.thesanctuary.co.uk/jordan
The best place for all therapies connected with the Dead Sea

Rosmoney Spa
Westport
County Mayo
Ireland
+ 353 98 28899
Thalassotherapy including sea-water swimming pool, seaweed treatments, thermal treatments, massage and meditation

Chiva Som
Hua Hin
Thailand
+ 66 32 536536
www.chivasom.net
Thai massage, meditation, t'ai chi, hydrotherapy

NORTHERN ITALY

In the Emilia-Romagna area around Parma in northern Italy are a number of spas that are based on the natural hot volcanic thermal springs in the area. Treatments include hydrotherapy, pools and steam grottos (in natural caves), mud therapies and vinotherapy (wine therapy). Three of the best are:

Grand Hotel Terme
Via Firenze, 15
48025 Riolo Terme (RA)
Italy
+ 39 546 71041

Terme della Salvarola
Hotel Salvarola Terme
41049
Sassuolo (MO)
Italy
+ 39 536 871788
www.termesalvarola.it
Terme de Salsomaggiore
Via Roma, 9
43039 Salsomaggiore (PR)
Italy
+ 39 524 578201

Index

Make
www.thorsonselement.com
your online sanctuary

Get online information, inspiration and
guidance to help you on the path to physical
and spiritual well-being. Drawing on the integrity
and vision of our authors and titles, and with
health advice, articles, astrology, tarot, a
meditation zone, author interviews and events
listings, www.thorsonselement.com is a great
alternative to help create space and peace
in our lives.

So if you've always wondered about practising
yoga, following an allergy-free diet, using the
tarot or getting a life coach, we can point you
in the right direction.

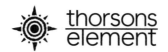